The Multi-Omics Revolution

Decoding Life with Multi-Omics

W J Francis

Copyright © 2024 by W J Francis

All rights reserved. No part of this book may be reproduced, distributed, or transmitted in any form or by any means, including photocopying, recording, or other electronic or mechanical methods, without the prior written permission of the publisher, except in the case of brief quotations embodied in critical reviews and certain other noncommercial uses permitted by copyright law.

DEDICATION

To the bright minds and hardworking hands building the future of technology. Your ingenuity, perseverance, and passion are what propel the contemporary world. This book honors your dedication to achieving the impossible.

Disclaimer: The information contained in this book is for educational and informational purposes only. It is not intended as medical advice and should not be relied upon as such. The author and publisher are not responsible for any adverse effects or consequences resulting from the use of any information, suggestions, or recommendations in this book

The Multi-Omics Revolution is a revolutionary movement that is changing our knowledge of life itself in the quickly changing fields of science and medicine.

This groundbreaking book reveals how the fields of genomics, proteomics, metabolomics, and more are combining to reshape technology, health, and our future. It takes you on an exciting trip through these interwoven fields.

Discover the power of multi-omics to unlock the secrets of human biology, tackle diseases with precision, and pioneer personalized medicine.

This book demonstrates how scientists and innovators are dismantling silos to produce a comprehensive picture of life's intricacies through engrossing tales, state-of-the-art research, and colorful explanations.

The Multi-Omics Revolution is the definitive resource for comprehending the technologies propelling the upcoming wave of innovations, written for inquisitive minds ranging from seasoned experts to ardent scientific lovers.

Whether you're intrigued by CRISPR's potential, fascinated by AI's role in decoding biology, or eager to explore how multi-omics is shaping fields from agriculture to climate science, this book is your roadmap to the future.

Join the revolution............

Explore the book that is redefining what is possible, igniting discussions, and inspiring discoveries.

With* The Multi-Omics Revolution, *the future isn't just near—it's already here.

W J Francis

CONTENTS

1. The Emergence of Multi-Omics 11

2. Scope and Importance of Single-Cell Multi-Omics 23

3. Principles of Single-Cell Biology 31

4. Technological Advances in Single-Cell Analysis 40

5. Omics Layers Explored 49

6. Methodologies for Multi-Omics Data Acquisition 70

7. Data Integration and Computational Tools 80

8. Standardization and Quality Control 90

9. Developmental Biology 99

10. Cancer Research 104

11. Neuroscience 113

12. Immunology 121

13. Regenerative Medicine 130

14. Microbiome Studies 139

15. Overcoming Technical and Analytical Challenges 148

16. Ethical and Privacy Considerations 157

17. Future Horizons in Single-Cell Multi-Omics 161

18. Revolutionizing Biology and Medicine 169

References 178

1. The Emergence of Multi-Omics

Historical Perspective on Omics Technologies

The journey of omics technologies traces back to the mid-20th century when scientists first began exploring the molecular underpinnings of life. This fascinating field has evolved dramatically over the decades, with each breakthrough shaping how we understand biology, medicine, and the environment. The term "omics" encompasses a broad range of scientific disciplines focused on studying and analyzing various biomolecules, such as genes, proteins, and metabolites, in a holistic manner.

The historical development of omics technologies offers insights into how interdisciplinary innovation has revolutionized our capacity to decipher life's complexity.

The Foundation: The DNA Revolution

The historical roots of omics technologies lie in the discovery of DNA's structure in 1953 by James Watson and Francis Crick, building on Rosalind Franklin's pivotal X-ray diffraction data. This milestone established the molecular basis of heredity, providing the foundation for genomics. The 1970s brought the advent of DNA sequencing, notably Fred Sanger's dideoxy sequencing method, which enabled scientists to determine the precise sequence of nucleotides in DNA.

This period also witnessed the birth of recombinant DNA technology, which allowed researchers to manipulate and study genes in unprecedented ways.

The Multi-Omics Revolution

The Rise of Genomics

Genomics, the first and most established omics field, began to take shape in the late 1980s. The Human Genome Project (HGP), initiated in 1990, was a landmark endeavor aimed at sequencing the entire human genome. This monumental project, completed in 2003, marked the beginning of the genomics revolution. The data it generated served as a blueprint for understanding genetic contributions to health and disease. Advances in sequencing technologies, such as next-generation sequencing (NGS), have since made genomic analyses faster, cheaper, and more accessible, driving discoveries across biology and medicine.

Expanding Beyond Genes: Transcriptomics

While genomics provided a static view of genetic material, transcriptomics emerged to study the dynamic expression of genes. The late 1990s saw the development of microarrays, a powerful tool for measuring gene expression across thousands of genes simultaneously. This technology was later surpassed by RNA sequencing (RNA-Seq), which provided more accurate and comprehensive data. Transcriptomics illuminated how genes are turned on or off in different conditions, revealing the intricate regulatory mechanisms that govern cellular function.

The Proteomics Revolution

Proteomics, the study of proteins, began gaining traction in the 1990s. Unlike DNA and RNA, proteins are the functional molecules that perform the tasks encoded by genes. Techniques like mass spectrometry (MS) and two-dimensional gel electrophoresis became cornerstones of proteomics, enabling the identification and quantification of proteins in complex samples. Proteomics has been instrumental in uncovering cellular processes, signaling pathways, and biomarkers for diseases, emphasizing the importance of proteins in understanding biological systems.

Entering the Metabolic World: Metabolomics

Metabolomics, focusing on small molecules and metabolites, arose in the early 2000s. These molecules are direct products of biochemical reactions, providing a snapshot of cellular activity. Advanced analytical techniques, such as nuclear magnetic resonance (NMR) spectroscopy and MS, allowed scientists to profile metabolites with remarkable sensitivity. Metabolomics has offered new perspectives on physiology, disease mechanisms, and the effects of environmental factors on biological systems.

The Emergence of Multi-Omics

The limitations of studying individual omics layers in isolation became evident as researchers sought to understand complex biological systems. The early 2010s marked the rise of multi-omics approaches, integrating genomics, transcriptomics, proteomics, metabolomics, and epigenomics.

This integration enabled a more comprehensive view of biological processes, capturing interactions between molecular layers. Multi-omics has been pivotal in systems biology, personalized medicine, and precision agriculture, offering holistic solutions to intricate scientific problems.

Technological Catalysts

Key technological innovations have driven the evolution of omics. The miniaturization of instruments, advances in computational power, and the development of sophisticated algorithms for data analysis have been crucial. Cloud computing and artificial intelligence now play significant roles in managing and interpreting the massive datasets generated by omics studies.

These advancements have made omics accessible to a broader range of researchers and industries.

The Multi-Omics Revolution

Societal Impact and Future Directions

The historical development of omics technologies has profoundly impacted science, healthcare, and agriculture. Genomic medicine, for instance, has revolutionized cancer treatment and rare disease diagnosis.

Multi-omics approaches are uncovering new drug targets, advancing understanding of microbiomes, and improving crop resilience.

Looking ahead, the integration of omics with emerging fields like synthetic biology and single-cell technologies promises to deepen our grasp of life's complexity.

The history of omics technologies is a testament to human curiosity and ingenuity. From the discovery of DNA's structure to the modern multi-omics era, this journey reflects an ongoing quest to unravel the mysteries of life, paving the way for a healthier, more sustainable future.

Why Single-Cell Analysis Matters

In recent years, single-cell analysis has emerged as one of the most transformative tools in modern biology and medicine.

Unlike traditional methods that study bulk populations of cells, single-cell analysis focuses on individual cells, enabling scientists to uncover the intricate complexities of cellular behavior, genetics, and interactions.

This granular approach offers unparalleled insights into biological systems, addressing questions that bulk analysis could never answer.

Let's explore why single-cell analysis matters and how it is revolutionizing science.

The Limitations of Bulk Analysis

Bulk cell analysis has been a cornerstone of biological research for decades, offering valuable insights into cellular processes. However, these methods average the signals from thousands or even millions of cells. This can obscure critical information, especially in heterogeneous cell populations, such as those found in tumors, the immune system, or developing embryos.

In bulk analysis, the unique characteristics of rare or distinct cell types are lost in the "average" data.

For example, imagine trying to understand a symphony by listening to all the instruments play together as one sound, without isolating each instrument. While the melody is clear, the contribution of individual instruments remains a mystery. Single-cell analysis breaks this barrier by "isolating the instruments," enabling researchers to study each cell's unique contribution.

Understanding Cellular Heterogeneity

No two cells are identical. Even within a seemingly uniform tissue, individual cells can differ in their gene expression, protein levels, metabolism, and function. These differences, known as cellular heterogeneity, are crucial in health and disease. Single-cell analysis provides a powerful lens to study this diversity.

For instance, in cancer, tumors often consist of a mosaic of different cell types. Some cells may be resistant to treatment, while others are more aggressive. By studying individual tumor cells, researchers can identify these subpopulations, uncovering mechanisms of drug resistance and paving the way for targeted therapies.

Similarly, in immunology, single-cell analysis reveals the diverse repertoire of immune cells, helping to design personalized vaccines and therapies.

The Multi-Omics Revolution

Unraveling Developmental Processes

Organismal development is a dynamic process where cells undergo numerous changes in function and identity. Single-cell analysis enables scientists to map these changes with unprecedented resolution.

By studying the gene expression profiles of individual cells at various stages of development, researchers can construct detailed "cellular atlases" that chart how cells differentiate and specialize.

For example, single-cell RNA sequencing has been used to map the development of human embryos, revealing the precise timing and sequence of gene activation that guides cell fate decisions.

This information is invaluable for understanding congenital disorders and improving regenerative medicine approaches, such as stem cell therapies.

Deciphering Complex Diseases

Complex diseases, such as neurodegenerative disorders, diabetes, and autoimmune conditions, often involve multiple cell types and intricate molecular interactions. Single-cell analysis allows researchers to dissect these interactions at an unparalleled level of detail.

In Alzheimer's disease, for example, single-cell analysis has identified specific brain cell populations that are more vulnerable to damage, shedding light on the early stages of disease progression. In diabetes research, this technology has revealed the diversity of pancreatic beta cells, offering clues about why some cells fail to produce insulin effectively.

These insights are driving the development of novel treatments tailored to individual cellular behaviors.

Advancing Precision Medicine

One of the most exciting applications of single-cell analysis is its role in precision medicine. By profiling individual cells, clinicians can identify unique biomarkers, predict patient responses to treatment, and monitor disease progression at a cellular level.

This is especially valuable in oncology, where understanding the genetic and molecular makeup of a patient's tumor can guide personalized treatment strategies.

Moreover, single-cell technologies are enabling the development of advanced immunotherapies, such as CAR-T cell therapy. By analyzing immune cells at a single-cell resolution, scientists can engineer therapies that are more effective and less toxic.

Driving Innovation in Multi-Omics

Single-cell analysis is not limited to studying just one type of data, such as gene expression. Recent advances have integrated multiple "omics" layers—genomics, transcriptomics, proteomics, epigenomics—within single cells. This multi-omics approach provides a comprehensive view of cellular function, linking genetic information to protein activity and cellular behavior. Such insights are driving discoveries in areas ranging from cancer biology to regenerative medicine.

The Future of Single-Cell Analysis

The rapid evolution of single-cell technologies, including single-cell RNA sequencing, mass cytometry, and spatial transcriptomics, is transforming biology. As these methods become more accessible and scalable, their applications are expanding into areas like drug discovery, agriculture, and environmental science.

Single-cell analysis is not just a tool; it is a paradigm shift, redefining how we study and understand life.

Single-cell analysis matters because it empowers us to study biology at its most fundamental level—the individual cell. By revealing the hidden heterogeneity within tissues, mapping developmental trajectories, and unraveling the complexities of disease, this technology is paving the way for breakthroughs in science and medicine. As the field continues to evolve, single-cell analysis will undoubtedly play a central role in addressing some of humanity's most pressing biological challenges.

Overview of Multi-Omics Integration

The field of life sciences is undergoing a profound transformation, driven by the rapid advancements in multi-omics technologies. Multi-omics refers to the integrated analysis of various "omics" layers, such as genomics, transcriptomics, proteomics, metabolomics, and epigenomics, to comprehensively understand biological systems. By combining insights from these individual layers, multi-omics integration provides a holistic view of the intricate molecular mechanisms underlying health, disease, and other biological processes.

The Need for Multi-Omics Integration
Traditional approaches in biology often focus on a single layer, such as the genome or transcriptome, to uncover insights into a biological system. However, biological systems are inherently complex and influenced by dynamic interactions across multiple layers. For example, while genomics provides the blueprint of an organism, the actual expression of genes (transcriptomics), the proteins they produce (proteomics), and the metabolic outcomes (metabolomics) all contribute to the phenotype. Studying each layer in isolation can miss critical interactions and fail to capture the complete picture.

Multi-omics integration addresses this limitation by bringing together data from various layers to create a comprehensive and interconnected understanding.

Key Components of Multi-Omics

Genomics: The study of the complete set of DNA, including genes and regulatory elements, forms the foundation of multi-omics. Genomics provides insights into genetic variations, mutations, and predispositions to diseases.

Transcriptomics: This layer focuses on RNA molecules transcribed from the genome, reflecting which genes are active and under what conditions. It helps link genetic information to functional outcomes.

Proteomics: Proteins are the functional molecules in a cell, responsible for structural, enzymatic, and signaling roles. Proteomics reveals how genes and transcripts translate into biological functions.

Metabolomics: The study of small molecules and metabolites provides a snapshot of biochemical activities, offering a dynamic view of cellular processes and physiological states.

Epigenomics: This layer examines heritable changes in gene expression that do not involve alterations in the DNA sequence, such as DNA methylation and histone modifications.

Challenges in Multi-Omics Integration

Integrating data from multiple omics layers is a challenging task due to the sheer volume, complexity, and heterogeneity of data. Each layer operates on different scales and employs unique measurement techniques.

For example, sequencing-based methods are common in genomics and transcriptomics, while mass spectrometry dominates proteomics and metabolomics.

Additionally, the biological interactions across these layers are nonlinear and context-dependent, making it difficult to build predictive models.

The Multi-Omics Revolution

Data integration also demands sophisticated computational tools and statistical methods.

Managing and analyzing multi-omics datasets require expertise in bioinformatics, machine learning, and systems biology.

Ensuring data quality, handling missing values, and overcoming batch effects further complicate the process.

Strategies for Multi-Omics Integration

Several computational and analytical approaches have been developed to integrate multi-omics data effectively:

Horizontal Integration: This involves combining data from the same omics layer across multiple samples or conditions. For instance, comparing gene expression profiles across different tissues or time points.

Vertical Integration: This strategy combines data from different omics layers for the same set of samples to understand cross-layer interactions.

For example, linking genetic variants with protein abundance and metabolite levels.

Network-Based Approaches: Biological networks, such as gene regulatory networks or protein-protein interaction networks, provide a framework to connect multi-omics data.

These approaches can identify key regulators or pathways driving a biological process.

Machine Learning Models: Advanced machine learning techniques, including deep learning and ensemble methods, are increasingly used to extract meaningful patterns from multi-omics datasets and predict outcomes such as disease risk or treatment response.

Applications of Multi-Omics Integration

The integration of multi-omics data has transformative implications across various fields:

Personalized Medicine: Multi-omics provides a detailed molecular profile of patients, enabling precise diagnosis, tailored treatments, and the identification of biomarkers for disease prediction.

Drug Discovery: Understanding how genetic, transcriptomic, proteomic, and metabolic changes interact can reveal new therapeutic targets and improve drug efficacy and safety assessments.

Agricultural Biotechnology: Multi-omics approaches are applied to improve crop yield, stress resistance, and nutritional value by understanding the underlying genetic and metabolic networks.

Environmental Sciences: Multi-omics helps study microbial communities, biogeochemical cycles, and ecosystem responses to environmental changes.

The Future of Multi-Omics Integration

As technology continues to advance, multi-omics integration is becoming more accessible and powerful.

High-throughput technologies, improved computational tools, and decreasing costs are enabling researchers to tackle complex questions at unprecedented scales.

The development of standardized data formats, cloud-based platforms, and collaborative efforts is further enhancing the usability of multi-omics approaches.

Looking ahead, multi-omics integration is expected to play a central role in systems biology, unraveling the complexities of life in greater detail.

The Multi-Omics Revolution

It holds promise not only for understanding disease mechanisms but also for solving global challenges such as food security and climate change.

By embracing the multi-omics revolution, scientists are poised to unlock new dimensions of discovery and innovation.

2. Scope and Importance of Single-Cell Multi-Omics

Addressing Cellular Heterogeneity

Cellular heterogeneity refers to the variation in cellular properties such as structure, function, gene expression, and response to stimuli within a population of cells, even when they originate from the same tissue or organism. This complexity poses challenges in understanding biological processes and developing targeted medical therapies, as traditional bulk analysis methods often mask the distinct contributions of individual cell types or states.

The advent of multi-omics technologies has revolutionized the study of cellular heterogeneity, enabling scientists to delve deeper into the intricate mosaic of life at an unprecedented resolution.

The Importance of Understanding Cellular Heterogeneity

Cells are not uniform entities; they differ in their roles, behaviors, and responses based on their environment and genetic programming. This variability is critical for physiological functions like immune responses, tissue repair, and development. However, it also plays a significant role in pathological contexts such as cancer, where subpopulations of tumor cells can drive drug resistance, metastasis, and recurrence.

Addressing cellular heterogeneity is, therefore, essential for advancing personalized medicine, refining diagnostic tools, and creating effective treatment strategies.

The Multi-Omics Revolution

Multi-Omics Approaches in Addressing Heterogeneity

Multi-omics integrates data from various omic layers—genomics, transcriptomics, proteomics, epigenomics, and metabolomics—to provide a comprehensive view of cellular states. By analyzing these data at the single-cell level, researchers can unravel the diversity within cell populations.

Single-Cell Genomics

Single-cell genomics allows for the exploration of genetic variations within individual cells. This is particularly useful for identifying mutations in cancer cells or tracing lineage relationships in developmental biology. Techniques like single-cell whole-genome sequencing and targeted gene panels have illuminated the mosaicism present in tissues, helping to differentiate between healthy and diseased states.

Single-Cell Transcriptomics

RNA sequencing (scRNA-seq) at the single-cell level measures gene expression profiles in individual cells, revealing functional differences that may not align with genetic changes. scRNA-seq has been instrumental in identifying rare cell types, such as stem cell subpopulations or immune cells responding to infection, and in constructing detailed cell atlases of tissues like the brain or liver.

Proteomics and Metabolomics

Proteins and metabolites are the direct effectors of cellular function, and their analysis complements genomics and transcriptomics. Single-cell proteomics technologies, like mass spectrometry and antibody-based assays, have provided insights into signaling pathways and post-translational modifications, which are crucial for understanding functional heterogeneity. Similarly, single-cell metabolomics uncovers metabolic adaptations in cancer cells or immune responses.

Spatial Multi-Omics

Spatially resolved technologies add an additional layer of information by preserving the context of cells within tissues. Methods like spatial transcriptomics and imaging mass cytometry combine single-cell data with tissue architecture, enabling researchers to understand how cellular heterogeneity contributes to tissue function and pathology. For instance, spatial analysis can reveal how tumor cells interact with the surrounding microenvironment, influencing progression and therapy resistance.

Advances in Computational Tools

The explosion of data generated by multi-omics requires sophisticated computational methods to integrate and interpret. Machine learning and artificial intelligence (AI) have emerged as indispensable tools in addressing cellular heterogeneity. These algorithms can identify patterns, classify cell types, and predict functional outcomes based on multi-dimensional datasets. Integrative frameworks, such as those combining transcriptomic and epigenomic data, have been used to map cellular trajectories during development or disease progression.

Applications in Medicine

Addressing cellular heterogeneity has profound implications for medicine.

Cancer Research: Multi-omics approaches have identified resistant subpopulations within tumors, guiding the development of combination therapies. Tumor heterogeneity studies also aid in understanding clonal evolution and metastasis.

Immune Therapies: By characterizing immune cell diversity, researchers have optimized immunotherapies such as CAR-T cells. Understanding how immune cells vary across individuals enhances vaccine development.

Regenerative Medicine: Single-cell analyses of stem cells provide insights into their differentiation potential, aiding in the design of regenerative therapies for degenerative diseases.

Challenges and Future Directions

While multi-omics has transformed our ability to address cellular heterogeneity, challenges remain. The cost and technical complexity of single-cell analyses limit accessibility, particularly in clinical settings.

Moreover, integrating and interpreting multi-layered omics data require further advancements in computational biology and data-sharing frameworks.

Future innovations are expected to refine these technologies, making them more scalable, accurate, and accessible. The development of high-throughput single-cell platforms, improved spatial resolution, and advanced AI-driven analytics will further enhance our understanding of cellular diversity.

These advances promise to translate into better diagnostics, more precise therapies, and deeper insights into fundamental biology.

The study of cellular heterogeneity is crucial for unraveling the complexities of life. Through multi-omics, researchers can dissect the intricate interplay of genetic, epigenetic, transcriptomic, proteomic, and metabolic layers in individual cells.

This integrated approach is not just a scientific endeavor but a cornerstone of personalized medicine, addressing the unique needs of each patient by understanding the fundamental variations within their cellular landscape.

As technologies continue to evolve, our ability to address cellular heterogeneity will only expand, offering unprecedented opportunities to tackle the most challenging questions in biology and medicine.

Transformative Impact on Biology and Medicine

The field of biology and medicine has witnessed groundbreaking advancements over the past few decades, but few have been as transformative as the advent of multi-omics technologies. This integrated approach, which combines various "omics" disciplines such as genomics, transcriptomics, proteomics, metabolomics, and epigenomics, has reshaped our understanding of life at a molecular level.

By examining the interplay of genes, proteins, metabolites, and their regulatory mechanisms, multi-omics provides a holistic view of biological systems.

This comprehensive perspective has revolutionized research and clinical practices, paving the way for personalized medicine, improved disease diagnostics, and novel therapeutic strategies.

From Reductionism to Systems Biology
Traditional biological studies often relied on a reductionist approach, focusing on isolated components such as single genes or proteins. While this methodology provided valuable insights, it fell short of capturing the complexity of living systems, where countless molecular interactions influence cellular and organismal behavior.

Multi-omics overcomes this limitation by adopting a systems biology perspective, integrating data from multiple layers of biological information.

This approach allows scientists to map intricate networks and identify patterns that were previously hidden.

By connecting the dots between various biological molecules, researchers can better understand the root causes of diseases and identify potential points of intervention.

Personalized and Precision Medicine

The Multi-Omics Revolution

One of the most profound impacts of the multi-omics revolution has been in the realm of personalized medicine. By analyzing a patient's genome, transcriptome, proteome, and metabolome, clinicians can gain a detailed understanding of their unique biological makeup. This enables the development of tailored treatment plans that account for individual variations, maximizing efficacy while minimizing side effects.

For instance, cancer therapies have greatly benefited from multi-omics approaches. Comprehensive profiling of tumors allows for the identification of specific genetic mutations, signaling pathways, and metabolic changes, leading to targeted therapies that improve patient outcomes.

Additionally, multi-omics has played a pivotal role in pharmacogenomics, the study of how genetic and molecular variations influence drug responses. By integrating omics data, researchers can predict adverse drug reactions, optimize dosing regimens, and identify novel drug targets, ultimately improving patient safety and therapeutic success.

Advancing Disease Diagnostics and Biomarker Discovery

Diagnosing complex diseases has historically been a challenge due to their multifactorial nature and the lack of reliable biomarkers. Multi-omics technologies have transformed this landscape by enabling the discovery of biomarkers across multiple molecular layers. For example, combining genomic and proteomic data can reveal genetic predispositions and protein expression changes associated with specific diseases. Metabolomics and lipidomics further add to this diagnostic arsenal by identifying alterations in metabolic pathways.

Such integrative biomarker discovery has led to earlier and more accurate diagnoses of diseases ranging from neurodegenerative disorders to cardiovascular conditions.

For example, in Alzheimer's disease, multi-omics approaches have identified molecular signatures that distinguish early stages of the disease, allowing for timely interventions. Similarly, in infectious diseases, multi-omics analyses of host-pathogen interactions have unveiled critical insights into immune responses and potential therapeutic targets.

Unraveling Complex Diseases

Many diseases, such as diabetes, cancer, and autoimmune disorders, arise from a combination of genetic, environmental, and lifestyle factors. Multi-omics has been instrumental in disentangling these complexities by providing a multidimensional view of disease mechanisms. By integrating genomic data with transcriptomic and epigenomic information, scientists can identify how genetic variants influence gene expression and epigenetic modifications. Proteomic and metabolomic data then shed light on downstream effects, such as altered protein functions and disrupted metabolic pathways.

This integrative approach has been particularly impactful in oncology. For instance, multi-omics studies have revealed distinct molecular subtypes of cancers, each with unique genetic alterations, protein expression profiles, and metabolic characteristics. These findings have redefined cancer classification systems and informed the development of subtype-specific treatments, improving patient prognoses.

Driving Innovations in Therapeutics

Beyond diagnostics and personalized medicine, multi-omics has accelerated therapeutic innovation. By providing a comprehensive understanding of disease biology, it has enabled the identification of novel drug targets and pathways. High-throughput omics technologies allow for the rapid screening of compounds, speeding up the drug discovery process. Moreover, multi-omics data is increasingly being used to inform the design of combination therapies, which target multiple pathways simultaneously for enhanced efficacy.

The Multi-Omics Revolution

For example, in autoimmune diseases, multi-omics analyses have identified shared and distinct molecular pathways underlying different conditions, guiding the development of drugs with broader or more specific therapeutic applications. Similarly, in rare genetic disorders, integrative omics approaches have uncovered disease-causing mutations and pathways, offering hope for targeted gene therapies.

The Future of Multi-Omics in Medicine

As multi-omics technologies continue to advance, their potential to transform biology and medicine grows exponentially. Emerging tools, such as single-cell omics and spatial omics, provide unprecedented resolution, allowing researchers to study molecular interactions at the level of individual cells and within their spatial context.

Additionally, advances in artificial intelligence and machine learning are enhancing the analysis of large and complex omics datasets, uncovering patterns and relationships that were previously inaccessible.

The integration of multi-omics data into clinical practice holds the promise of predictive healthcare, where diseases can be prevented or mitigated before they manifest.

Furthermore, as multi-omics becomes more accessible and cost-effective, its benefits will extend to broader populations, reducing healthcare disparities and improving global health outcomes.

In conclusion, the multi-omics revolution has profoundly impacted biology and medicine, shifting paradigms and unlocking new possibilities.

By bridging the gap between molecular complexity and clinical application, it has laid the foundation for a future where precision, personalization, and prevention are the cornerstones of healthcare.

3. Principles of Single-Cell Biology

Cellular Heterogeneity in Development and Disease

Cellular heterogeneity refers to the diversity of cells within a population, even among cells that are seemingly identical in type and function. This phenomenon plays a pivotal role in both the development of organisms and the progression of diseases. Advances in the field of multi-omics have revolutionized our ability to study cellular heterogeneity, offering profound insights into how individual cells contribute to the complexity of life and how they influence health and disease.

Cellular Heterogeneity in Development

During development, a single fertilized egg undergoes numerous divisions and differentiations, giving rise to the trillions of specialized cells in an organism. Cellular heterogeneity is fundamental to this process. It enables the formation of diverse cell types, such as neurons, muscle cells, and immune cells, each with unique functions.

This heterogeneity is orchestrated by tightly regulated processes involving gene expression, epigenetic modifications, and environmental signals. For example, stem cells, which are undifferentiated cells capable of giving rise to various cell types, exhibit heterogeneity in their gene expression profiles.

This variability allows them to respond dynamically to developmental cues, choosing specific pathways of differentiation based on their microenvironment.

The Multi-Omics Revolution

Recent multi-omics approaches, which integrate genomics, transcriptomics, proteomics, and epigenomics, have unveiled the intricate networks underlying cellular heterogeneity. By analyzing single-cell data, researchers can map how different cells transition from one state to another during development.

Such studies have revealed previously unknown intermediate states, providing a more nuanced understanding of developmental biology.

Cellular Heterogeneity in Disease

Cellular heterogeneity is equally crucial in understanding disease, particularly complex conditions like cancer, neurodegenerative disorders, and infectious diseases. In cancer, for instance, a tumor is rarely a uniform mass of identical cells. Instead, it consists of a heterogeneous population of cancer cells with distinct genetic mutations, metabolic profiles, and resistance to treatments.

This heterogeneity makes it challenging to treat cancer effectively, as therapies targeting one subpopulation may leave others unaffected.

Similarly, in neurodegenerative diseases like Alzheimer's, cellular heterogeneity among neurons and glial cells contributes to disease progression. Some cells are more vulnerable to damage, while others might exhibit protective responses. Understanding this diversity can guide the development of targeted therapies aimed at preserving or restoring normal cellular functions.

In infectious diseases, heterogeneity among immune cells determines the effectiveness of the body's response. For example, during a viral infection, some T cells might mount a strong immune response, while others remain inactive. This variability can influence the severity of the disease and the success of treatments like vaccines.

The Role of Multi-Omics in Studying Cellular Heterogeneity

The advent of multi-omics technologies has transformed our ability to study cellular heterogeneity in unprecedented detail. Single-cell sequencing, for example, allows researchers to analyze the genetic and transcriptomic profiles of individual cells, revealing subtle differences that were previously undetectable in bulk analyses.

Epigenomic studies uncover variations in DNA modifications and chromatin accessibility, which regulate gene expression without altering the genetic code. Proteomic analyses provide insights into the diverse proteins expressed by cells, while metabolomics sheds light on the biochemical pathways that vary between cell populations.

Integrating these layers of information enables a holistic view of cellular heterogeneity. For example, combining transcriptomics and epigenomics can reveal how changes in chromatin structure influence gene expression in specific cell types. Such insights are invaluable for understanding how cellular states evolve during development or disease progression.

Implications for Medicine and Therapeutics

Recognizing and studying cellular heterogeneity have profound implications for medicine. In cancer treatment, for instance, identifying distinct subpopulations of tumor cells can inform the design of combination therapies that target multiple pathways simultaneously. This approach can overcome resistance and improve patient outcomes.

In regenerative medicine, understanding the heterogeneity of stem cells is critical for developing effective therapies. Researchers can harness this knowledge to optimize the differentiation of stem cells into desired cell types, ensuring their successful integration into damaged tissues.

The Multi-Omics Revolution

In infectious diseases, analyzing the heterogeneity of immune responses can guide vaccine development. For example, identifying the characteristics of immune cells that mount effective responses can inform the design of vaccines that elicit similar protective immunity.

Future Directions

The study of cellular heterogeneity is still in its infancy, but the rapid advancement of multi-omics technologies promises an exciting future.

Emerging tools, such as spatial transcriptomics and advanced imaging techniques, allow researchers to study cells in their native tissue environments.

This spatial context is crucial for understanding how cells interact with each other and with their surroundings.

Furthermore, the integration of multi-omics data with machine learning is opening new avenues for discovering patterns in cellular heterogeneity.

These approaches can help predict how cells will behave in response to specific stimuli, enabling more precise interventions in both development and disease.

In conclusion, cellular heterogeneity is a cornerstone of biology, driving the complexity of development and influencing the progression of diseases.

The multi-omics revolution has provided powerful tools to unravel this complexity, offering new insights into the dynamic nature of cells.

By continuing to explore cellular heterogeneity, we can pave the way for transformative advancements in science and medicine.

Concepts of Systems Biology

Systems biology is a groundbreaking approach to understanding life by examining the interactions and relationships between components of biological systems.

Unlike traditional biology, which often focuses on studying individual parts such as genes, proteins, or cells in isolation, systems biology emphasizes the whole system, considering how these parts work together to create the dynamic processes of life.

By integrating data from multiple disciplines, systems biology provides a more holistic understanding of biological functions and their underlying mechanisms.

The Shift from Reductionism to Holism

For much of the history of biology, scientists have relied on a reductionist approach, breaking down organisms into their smallest parts to study them in detail.

While this method has led to significant discoveries, it often fails to capture the complexity of how components interact within a living organism.

Systems biology takes a holistic perspective, aiming to understand the emergent properties—behaviors and functions that arise from the collective interactions of system components.

Emergent properties cannot be predicted merely by examining individual parts. For example, understanding a single neuron's function does not reveal how a network of neurons produces cognition or consciousness.

Systems biology focuses on deciphering these intricate interactions, leveraging computational models, advanced technologies, and interdisciplinary collaboration.

Key Principles of Systems Biology

Interconnectedness of Components

Biological systems are composed of interconnected components that interact to form a complex network. These interactions can be physical, such as protein-protein interactions, or functional, like gene regulation pathways. Understanding these networks is critical to identifying how disruptions in one part can lead to cascading effects, such as diseases.

Dynamic Behavior

Biological systems are dynamic and change over time in response to internal and external cues. Systems biology investigates these temporal changes, such as how gene expression varies during development, disease progression, or environmental stress. Time-series data and computational models help capture these dynamics, offering insights into the underlying regulatory mechanisms.

Multiscale Integration

Biological systems operate across multiple scales, from molecules to ecosystems. Systems biology seeks to integrate information across these scales, recognizing that changes at the molecular level can influence cellular behavior, tissue function, and even organismal health. For example, in cancer research, systems biology might connect mutations in DNA to changes in cell signaling pathways, leading to tumor growth and metastasis.

Feedback and Regulation

Feedback loops, both positive and negative, are fundamental in maintaining homeostasis within biological systems. Systems biology examines these regulatory mechanisms to understand how stability and flexibility are achieved. For instance, negative feedback helps stabilize blood glucose levels, while positive feedback amplifies signals in processes like blood clotting.

Technologies Driving Systems Biology

The rise of systems biology has been fueled by technological advancements that generate large-scale data and enable its analysis.

Some of the key technologies include:

Omics Platforms: Genomics, transcriptomics, proteomics, metabolomics, and epigenomics provide comprehensive data about the different molecular layers in a system.

High-Throughput Sequencing: Allows the rapid analysis of entire genomes and transcriptomes, providing detailed insights into genetic and functional variations.

Mass Spectrometry and Imaging: Enable the study of proteins, metabolites, and cellular structures with high precision.

Bioinformatics and Computational Modeling: Advanced algorithms and software tools are essential for analyzing complex datasets, constructing models, and simulating biological processes.

Applications of Systems Biology

Medicine and Healthcare
Systems biology is transforming medicine by enabling personalized approaches to treatment.

For instance, in cancer, multi-omics data can help identify specific biomarkers and tailor therapies to an individual's unique molecular profile.

Similarly, systems biology aids in understanding complex diseases like diabetes or Alzheimer's by integrating genetic, metabolic, and environmental factors.

Drug Discovery

By mapping interaction networks and identifying key regulatory nodes, systems biology can reveal potential drug targets and predict off-target effects, accelerating the drug discovery process.

Synthetic Biology

Systems biology informs the design of synthetic biological systems, such as engineered microbes for producing biofuels or pharmaceuticals. Understanding natural system dynamics helps scientists construct artificial systems with desired properties.

Agriculture and Environmental Science

In agriculture, systems biology can enhance crop resilience by analyzing stress-response networks. In environmental science, it helps study microbial communities and their roles in ecosystems, such as carbon cycling or pollutant degradation.

Challenges and Future Directions

While systems biology has made remarkable strides, challenges remain. Integrating diverse datasets across multiple scales and types is computationally intensive and requires robust algorithms. Additionally, biological systems are inherently noisy and variable, complicating the development of predictive models.

The future of systems biology lies in its integration with emerging technologies such as artificial intelligence and quantum computing. These tools can enhance data analysis, improve model accuracy, and uncover new biological insights.

Collaborative efforts across disciplines will also be vital to fully realizing the potential of systems biology in addressing global challenges, from curing diseases to combating climate change.

Systems biology represents a paradigm shift in how we study life.

By focusing on the interactions and networks within biological systems, it provides a comprehensive understanding that goes beyond the sum of individual components.

This approach is unlocking new frontiers in science and medicine, promising innovative solutions to some of humanity's most pressing problems.

The multi-omics revolution is a cornerstone of this transformation, enabling systems biology to thrive in the era of big data and precision science.

4. Technological Advances in Single-Cell Analysis

Microfluidics and Sequencing Technologies

In the realm of modern biology, the advent of multi-omics—the integrated study of genomics, transcriptomics, proteomics, metabolomics, and other omics layers—has revolutionized our understanding of life. At the heart of this revolution lie two transformative technologies: microfluidics and sequencing technologies. Together, they provide the tools to analyze biological systems with unprecedented precision and depth.

Microfluidics: Miniaturizing Biology
Microfluidics involves the manipulation of tiny volumes of liquids, often at the scale of microliters or nanoliters, through channels and chambers no wider than a strand of hair. This technology, inspired by the miniaturization trends in electronics, has redefined biological experimentation.

Key Advantages of Microfluidics

Precision and Control: Microfluidics enables the manipulation of single cells and molecules, ensuring precise analysis of biological samples.

Reduced Sample and Reagent Use: By working with minuscule volumes, microfluidics minimizes waste, reducing the cost of reagents and allowing studies on limited or precious samples.

High Throughput: With automated systems and parallel processing, microfluidics can process thousands of samples simultaneously, a crucial capability for large-scale omics studies.

Applications in Multi-Omics

In the context of multi-omics, microfluidics facilitates the isolation and analysis of individual components of biological systems:

Single-Cell Analysis: Traditional methods average data across millions of cells, masking cellular heterogeneity.

Microfluidics allows the isolation of individual cells, enabling the study of single-cell transcriptomes, epigenomes, and proteomes.

Proteomics and Metabolomics: Microfluidic chips can separate and quantify proteins and metabolites with extreme sensitivity, aiding in the exploration of cellular functions.

Integration Across Omics Layers: By miniaturizing and integrating workflows, microfluidic platforms support simultaneous analysis of multiple omics layers from the same sample.
For instance, a microfluidic device might isolate a single cell, lyse it to release its contents, and channel the DNA for sequencing, while proteins and metabolites are directed to other analytical modules.

This integration is essential for understanding the dynamic interplay between different molecular layers.

Sequencing Technologies: Reading the Blueprint of Life

Parallel to the rise of microfluidics, advancements in sequencing technologies have been equally transformative.

The ability to rapidly and accurately decode the genetic and epigenetic information of organisms has expanded our capacity to study life at its most fundamental level.

The Multi-Omics Revolution

The Evolution of Sequencing

Sanger Sequencing: Introduced in the 1970s, this method was a groundbreaking achievement but limited by its low throughput and high cost.

Next-Generation Sequencing (NGS): The early 21st century saw the advent of NGS, enabling massive parallel sequencing.

This leap drastically reduced the cost of sequencing, making it accessible for large-scale projects like the Human Genome Project.

Third-Generation and Beyond: Recent innovations, such as single-molecule sequencing and nanopore technology, have improved read lengths and real-time capabilities, broadening the applications of sequencing.

Applications in Multi-Omics

Sequencing technologies form the backbone of multi-omics by providing insights into various molecular layers:

Genomics: High-throughput sequencing deciphers entire genomes, uncovering genetic variants and structural alterations.

Transcriptomics: RNA sequencing (RNA-Seq) measures gene expression, revealing how genes are turned on or off in specific contexts.

Epigenomics: Techniques like bisulfite sequencing and ATAC-Seq map DNA modifications and chromatin accessibility, shedding light on gene regulation.

Metagenomics: Sequencing enables the study of microbial communities, revealing the interplay between host and microbiome in health and disease.

Synergy Between Microfluidics and Sequencing

The integration of microfluidics with sequencing technologies amplifies the potential of multi-omics research. Microfluidic platforms streamline the preparation of sequencing libraries, reducing manual steps and potential errors. For instance:

Single-cell RNA sequencing relies on microfluidics to encapsulate individual cells in droplets, where they are lysed, and their RNA is barcoded for sequencing.

Microfluidic chips automate the enrichment and sorting of specific DNA or RNA fragments, enhancing the efficiency and resolution of sequencing analyses.

This synergy is particularly impactful in fields like cancer research, where understanding tumor heterogeneity requires high-resolution single-cell sequencing. It also drives innovations in personalized medicine, enabling tailored therapeutic strategies based on comprehensive multi-omics profiles.

Challenges and Future Directions

Despite their transformative impact, microfluidics and sequencing technologies face challenges:

Scalability: Expanding microfluidic platforms to handle larger sample sizes while maintaining precision is a technical hurdle.
Data Integration: Multi-omics studies generate vast, complex datasets, requiring advanced computational tools for integration and interpretation.

Cost: While costs have decreased, widespread adoption of cutting-edge technologies remains financially challenging for smaller laboratories.

Looking ahead, the field is poised for further innovations. Advances in materials science may produce more robust and versatile microfluidic devices.

The Multi-Omics Revolution

Meanwhile, sequencing technologies are trending toward faster, more accurate, and cost-effective solutions.

Together, these advancements will democratize access to multi-omics tools, empowering researchers worldwide.

The confluence of microfluidics and sequencing technologies has catalyzed the multi-omics revolution, unraveling the intricate web of molecular interactions that define life.

By enabling high-resolution, high-throughput analyses, these technologies provide the foundation for breakthroughs in biology, medicine, and beyond.

As we continue to refine and integrate these tools, the promise of multi-omics to transform our understanding of complex biological systems and improve human health grows ever brighter.

Challenges of Working at the Single-Cell Level

The study of biology has reached unprecedented precision with the advent of single-cell technologies.

By examining individual cells, scientists can unravel the intricate complexity of tissues, organs, and systems that were previously obscured by bulk-level analyses.

However, while single-cell research holds tremendous promise, it also presents significant technical, analytical, and logistical challenges.

These hurdles must be addressed to fully unlock the potential of single-cell multi-omics and revolutionize our understanding of life at its most granular level.

Sample Preparation and Cell Viability

One of the primary challenges in single-cell studies is the preparation of viable and representative samples. Cells are inherently fragile and susceptible to stress during isolation procedures. Techniques such as fluorescence-activated cell sorting (FACS) or microfluidics, while powerful, can introduce biases or damage, compromising the integrity of the cells and their molecular content. Additionally, certain cell types may be more challenging to isolate due to their physical properties or scarcity, making it difficult to achieve a truly representative dataset.

Low Biomolecular Content and Sensitivity Issues

Unlike bulk samples, where the molecular content of thousands of cells is averaged, single-cell studies analyze the minute quantities of DNA, RNA, proteins, and metabolites present in individual cells. This necessitates highly sensitive and precise detection methods, as even the slightest technical noise or contamination can significantly skew results. Amplification methods used to enhance these signals, such as PCR for DNA and RNA or mass spectrometry for metabolites, can inadvertently introduce biases, leading to a loss of quantitative accuracy.

Capturing Cellular Heterogeneity

While single-cell approaches aim to capture cellular heterogeneity, ensuring that this diversity is accurately represented poses another challenge. Biological samples often contain a wide array of cell types and states, and isolating rare or transient populations requires exceptional precision.

The process is further complicated by the dynamic nature of cells; their molecular profiles can change rapidly in response to environmental stimuli, making it difficult to capture a snapshot that reflects their true state.

Multi-Omic Integration

Single-cell multi-omics integrates various data layers, such as genomics, transcriptomics, proteomics, and metabolomics, from the same cell. While this holistic approach provides a comprehensive view of cellular function, it also amplifies complexity. Each omic layer requires specialized techniques and produces datasets with distinct characteristics and noise profiles. Integrating these diverse datasets to derive biologically meaningful insights demands advanced computational tools and robust experimental design.

Data Processing and Computational Challenges

Single-cell experiments generate massive amounts of data. A single run can produce terabytes of information that must be processed, analyzed, and stored. The high dimensionality of single-cell datasets necessitates specialized algorithms capable of handling sparsity and noise.

For example, dropout effects in single-cell RNA sequencing, where certain genes appear undetected due to technical limitations, must be carefully addressed to avoid misinterpretation. Additionally, computational tools must account for batch effects, which can arise from variations in experimental conditions and lead to artificial differences between samples.

Cost and Accessibility

Single-cell technologies remain expensive, both in terms of equipment and reagents. Platforms such as single-cell RNA sequencing or CyTOF (mass cytometry) require highly specialized instruments, consumables, and expertise.

This cost barrier limits access to single-cell research, particularly for labs in resource-constrained settings, potentially exacerbating disparities in scientific research globally.

Ethical and Regulatory Considerations

Single-cell studies often involve human tissues, raising ethical concerns about privacy and consent.

For instance, single-cell genomics can reveal detailed genetic information, including rare mutations, which could inadvertently identify individuals or their relatives.

Ensuring compliance with ethical guidelines and addressing potential regulatory challenges is crucial for responsible research.

Validation and Reproducibility

Validating findings in single-cell studies can be particularly challenging due to the inherent variability among individual cells and the low sample size in some experiments.

Reproducibility can also be a concern; results from one lab may not easily translate to another due to differences in protocols, equipment, or data analysis methods.

Standardization of workflows and robust benchmarking are essential to improve confidence in single-cell research outcomes.

Scaling and Throughput

As the field advances, the demand for high-throughput single-cell analyses continues to grow. Scaling these studies while maintaining accuracy and affordability is a significant challenge. Current technologies often involve labor-intensive and time-consuming steps, which limit their application to larger cohorts or longitudinal studies.

Developing automated and scalable solutions will be key to overcoming this limitation.

Future Directions and Solutions

Despite these challenges, ongoing advancements are poised to address many of these issues.

For example, innovations in microfluidics and droplet-based systems are improving cell capture and throughput. Novel amplification and sequencing technologies are enhancing sensitivity and reducing technical noise.

Computational biology is evolving rapidly, with machine learning and artificial intelligence driving progress in data integration and analysis.

Collaborative efforts among researchers, institutions, and industries are helping to reduce costs and democratize access to single-cell technologies.

In conclusion, while the challenges of working at the single-cell level are substantial, they are not insurmountable.

By developing robust methodologies, fostering interdisciplinary collaboration, and addressing ethical and accessibility concerns, the scientific community can continue to push the boundaries of what is possible in single-cell research.

This endeavor holds the promise of transforming our understanding of biology and paving the way for groundbreaking applications in medicine, biotechnology, and beyond.

5. Omics Layers Explored

Genomics: Single-Cell Genome Sequencing

The complexity of life is built upon the blueprint of DNA, and genomic technologies have revolutionized our ability to decipher this code.

Traditional genome sequencing has allowed us to understand the genetic makeup of organisms, but it often relies on pooling genetic material from millions of cells, masking the variability between individual cells.

Enter single-cell genome sequencing—a transformative approach that unveils the genetic identity of individual cells, offering unprecedented insights into cellular diversity, development, and disease.

What is Single-Cell Genome Sequencing?

Single-cell genome sequencing is a cutting-edge technique that deciphers the complete DNA sequence of an individual cell.

Unlike traditional methods that aggregate genetic information, this approach isolates a single cell, amplifies its DNA, and sequences it to generate a comprehensive genome profile.

This granular view reveals variations such as mutations, copy number alterations, and chromosomal rearrangements unique to each cell.

Why Single Cells?

Cells in a multicellular organism can differ significantly, even when they share the same genome.

This heterogeneity is critical for normal functions such as development, immune responses, and tissue repair.

However, it also plays a role in pathological conditions like cancer, where genetic variability within a tumor can drive drug resistance and metastasis.

By analyzing single cells, researchers can uncover hidden genomic differences that are essential for understanding biology and improving therapeutic strategies.

The Workflow of Single-Cell Genome Sequencing

The process begins with isolating individual cells from a tissue or biological sample.

Various techniques such as fluorescence-activated cell sorting (FACS), microfluidics, or manual micromanipulation are used for this purpose.

Once a single cell is isolated, its DNA is extracted and amplified to produce sufficient material for sequencing.

This amplification step, often performed using methods like multiple displacement amplification (MDA) or polymerase chain reaction (PCR), is crucial because a single cell contains a minuscule amount of DNA.

After amplification, the DNA is sequenced using next-generation sequencing (NGS) technologies, generating millions of short DNA reads.

Computational algorithms then assemble these reads into a complete genome, identifying genetic variants and structural changes.

Applications in Science and Medicine

Cancer Research:
Single-cell genome sequencing has become a powerful tool in oncology. Tumors are often composed of genetically diverse cell populations, and this heterogeneity is a major challenge in cancer treatment. By sequencing individual tumor cells, researchers can identify subpopulations with specific mutations, understand the mechanisms of metastasis, and design targeted therapies.

Developmental Biology:
In embryonic development, a single fertilized egg divides and differentiates into a multitude of specialized cell types. Single-cell genome sequencing helps trace the lineage of cells, revealing how genetic changes influence differentiation and tissue formation.

Neurological Disorders:
The brain is an exceptionally heterogeneous organ, with neurons and glial cells exhibiting diverse genomic profiles. Single-cell genome sequencing has been instrumental in studying conditions like Alzheimer's disease and schizophrenia, uncovering genetic anomalies at the cellular level that were previously undetectable.

Infectious Diseases:
Pathogens like viruses and bacteria can evolve rapidly within a host. Single-cell genome sequencing allows scientists to study these evolutionary dynamics by sequencing individual microbial cells or infected host cells, providing insights into drug resistance and immune evasion.

Reproductive Medicine:
In preimplantation genetic testing, single-cell genome sequencing is used to screen embryos for genetic disorders before implantation in in-vitro fertilization (IVF). This ensures a higher likelihood of healthy pregnancies and reduces the risk of inherited diseases.

The Multi-Omics Revolution

Challenges and Innovations

Despite its promise, single-cell genome sequencing faces several challenges. One major issue is amplification bias, where certain genomic regions are overrepresented or underrepresented during the DNA amplification step.

This can lead to incomplete or inaccurate sequencing data. Additionally, the technical difficulty of isolating single cells without contamination and the high cost of sequencing remain barriers to widespread adoption.

However, recent innovations are addressing these limitations. Advances in microfluidic technology have made cell isolation more efficient and scalable.

Improved amplification methods and error-correction algorithms are enhancing the accuracy of sequencing data.

Furthermore, the integration of single-cell genome sequencing with other multi-omics approaches, such as transcriptomics and epigenomics, is providing a more holistic view of cellular function.

Future Prospects

The future of single-cell genome sequencing is bright, with applications poised to expand across disciplines. In personalized medicine, the technique holds the potential to tailor treatments based on the unique genomic profile of an individual's cells.

In ecology and evolutionary biology, it can reveal the genetic diversity within microbial communities or track the evolution of species.

As costs decrease and technologies become more accessible, single-cell genome sequencing is set to become a cornerstone of biological research and clinical practice.

Single-cell genome sequencing represents a paradigm shift in genomics, enabling researchers to explore the genetic intricacies of life at an unprecedented resolution. By unraveling the DNA of individual cells, this technology is illuminating the cellular heterogeneity that underpins development, disease, and evolution. As innovations continue to refine its capabilities, single-cell genome sequencing will undoubtedly play a pivotal role in advancing science and improving human health.

This revolutionary approach not only deepens our understanding of biology but also paves the way for breakthroughs in diagnostics, therapeutics, and beyond.

Transcriptomics: Single-cell RNA-seq

Transcriptomics, the study of RNA transcripts within a cell, has been revolutionized by the advent of single-cell RNA sequencing (scRNA-seq). This groundbreaking technique enables researchers to delve into the gene expression profiles of individual cells, offering unprecedented insights into cellular diversity, function, and behavior. The ability to analyze the transcriptomes of thousands of cells simultaneously has transformed our understanding of complex biological systems and disease mechanisms.

The Basics of RNA and Gene Expression

RNA, or ribonucleic acid, is the molecule that carries genetic instructions from DNA to the protein-synthesizing machinery of the cell. These instructions dictate which proteins a cell produces, directly influencing its function. However, gene expression is not uniform across cells, even within the same tissue. Variations in RNA expression levels underlie cellular diversity and specialization. Understanding these differences is critical for deciphering biological complexity and addressing questions related to development, health, and disease.

The Multi-Omics Revolution

The Evolution of RNA Analysis

Traditional methods for studying gene expression, such as bulk RNA sequencing, provide an averaged view of transcriptomes across a population of cells.

While valuable, this approach masks the heterogeneity within a sample.

For example, rare cell types or transient states can be overlooked. Single-cell RNA sequencing overcomes this limitation by isolating and analyzing individual cells, revealing a high-resolution snapshot of gene expression dynamics.

How Single-cell RNA-seq Works

The process of scRNA-seq involves several key steps:

Cell Isolation: Individual cells are separated from a tissue or culture. Techniques such as fluorescence-activated cell sorting (FACS), microfluidic devices, or droplet-based methods are commonly used for this purpose.

RNA Capture and Conversion: Once isolated, the RNA within each cell is extracted and converted into complementary DNA (cDNA) through reverse transcription. This step is crucial because cDNA is more stable and can be amplified for sequencing.

Library Preparation and Sequencing: The cDNA is prepared for sequencing by adding adapters and barcodes that uniquely label the transcripts from each cell. High-throughput sequencing technologies are then used to generate massive amounts of data.

Data Analysis: The sequencing reads are aligned to a reference genome, and computational tools are used to quantify gene expression levels, identify cell types, and uncover functional states.

Applications of Single-cell RNA-seq

Understanding Cellular Heterogeneity: scRNA-seq has been instrumental in identifying previously unknown cell types and subtypes in various tissues, such as immune cells, neurons, and cancer cells. This knowledge is crucial for understanding tissue organization and function.

Developmental Biology: By capturing the transcriptomes of individual cells at different stages of development, researchers can reconstruct cell lineage trajectories and uncover the molecular events guiding differentiation.

Cancer Research: Tumors are highly heterogeneous, consisting of diverse cancer cell populations and surrounding stromal cells. scRNA-seq allows scientists to dissect this complexity, identify resistant subclones, and understand tumor evolution.

Immunology: The immune system comprises a diverse array of cell types that respond dynamically to infections and other challenges. scRNA-seq provides detailed maps of immune responses, aiding vaccine development and immunotherapy design.

Neurology: Single-cell RNA sequencing is shedding light on the intricate cellular composition of the brain, revealing new insights into neural development, function, and disorders like Alzheimer's and Parkinson's disease.

Advancements and Challenges

Recent advances in scRNA-seq have significantly improved its sensitivity, resolution, and scalability. Techniques like multi-modal single-cell profiling now integrate transcriptomic data with other molecular layers, such as epigenomics and proteomics, providing a holistic view of cellular states. Computational tools and machine learning approaches are also enhancing data interpretation, enabling researchers to uncover complex patterns and predict cellular behavior.

Despite these advancements, scRNA-seq faces challenges. The technique is resource-intensive, requiring sophisticated equipment and computational infrastructure. Additionally, the loss of spatial context during cell isolation can obscure interactions between cells and their microenvironment. Emerging methods like spatial transcriptomics are addressing this limitation by preserving tissue architecture while analyzing gene expression.

Transformative Potential

Single-cell RNA sequencing is not just a technological breakthrough—it represents a paradigm shift in biological research. By unraveling the molecular intricacies of individual cells, scRNA-seq empowers researchers to address questions that were previously inaccessible. From personalized medicine to regenerative therapies, the implications are profound and far reaching.

The Road Ahead

As scRNA-seq continues to evolve, its integration with other "omics" technologies will likely drive the next wave of discoveries. For example, combining transcriptomics with proteomics and metabolomics will provide a comprehensive understanding of cellular function. These advancements will undoubtedly pave the way for new diagnostics, therapeutics, and strategies to combat diseases at their roots.

In summary, single-cell RNA sequencing has revolutionized transcriptomics, offering an unparalleled window into the world of individual cells. Its ability to capture cellular diversity, unravel developmental pathways, and illuminate disease mechanisms underscores its transformative impact on science and medicine.

As we continue to push the boundaries of this technology, the possibilities for discovery are virtually limitless.

Epigenomics: Chromatin Accessibility and Methylation

Epigenomics represents a revolutionary lens through which we understand the regulation of gene expression without altering the underlying DNA sequence. At its core, epigenomics studies chemical modifications to DNA and its associated proteins that impact how genes are turned on or off. Two key aspects of this field are chromatin accessibility and DNA methylation—both essential for controlling cellular identity and function.

Chromatin Accessibility

DNA in our cells is tightly packed into a structure called chromatin. This packaging ensures that the nearly two meters of DNA in each cell fits within the microscopic nucleus. However, this compact arrangement also determines whether genes are accessible for transcription, the process by which genes are read and converted into RNA and proteins.

Chromatin exists in two primary states:

Euchromatin: Loosely packed and transcriptionally active, allowing genes in these regions to be readily accessed by transcription machinery.

Heterochromatin: Tightly packed and transcriptionally silent, where genes are typically inactive.

Chromatin accessibility is dynamically regulated by molecular complexes that modify histones (the proteins DNA wraps around) or reposition nucleosomes (DNA-protein complexes). Enzymes such as histone acetyltransferases (HATs) loosen chromatin by adding acetyl groups to histones, enhancing gene accessibility. Conversely, histone deacetylases (HDACs) remove these acetyl groups, compacting chromatin and silencing genes.

Techniques such as ATAC-seq (Assay for Transposase-Accessible Chromatin using sequencing) have been developed to study chromatin accessibility across the genome.

These technologies enable scientists to pinpoint regions of open chromatin, often correlating with active genes or regulatory elements like enhancers and promoters.

The findings provide critical insights into cell-specific gene regulation and how changes in chromatin accessibility contribute to diseases, including cancer.

DNA Methylation

DNA methylation is another cornerstone of epigenomics. It involves the addition of a methyl group ($-CH_3$) to cytosine bases in DNA, typically at CpG sites (where cytosine is followed by guanine). This modification generally represses gene expression, either by directly preventing transcription factors from binding to DNA or by recruiting proteins that compact chromatin into an inaccessible state.

During development, DNA methylation plays a crucial role in establishing cellular identity by ensuring that only the necessary genes for a particular cell type are active. For instance, methylation patterns differ markedly between neurons and muscle cells, even though they share the same genome.

DNA methylation is dynamic and reversible, allowing cells to respond to environmental cues. For example, dietary factors, stress, or toxins can alter methylation patterns, influencing health outcomes. Abnormal DNA methylation is often implicated in diseases:

Hypermethylation at tumor suppressor genes can silence their protective effects, contributing to cancer development.
Hypomethylation can activate oncogenes or destabilize the genome, further promoting malignancy.

Advanced sequencing technologies like whole-genome bisulfite sequencing (WGBS) allow researchers to map DNA methylation at single-base resolution. These tools have uncovered intricate methylation landscapes in various tissues and disease states, paving the way for diagnostic and therapeutic applications.

Interplay Between Chromatin Accessibility and Methylation

Although chromatin accessibility and DNA methylation are distinct mechanisms, they often work in concert. Open chromatin regions are typically associated with low DNA methylation and active gene expression. Conversely, closed chromatin is enriched with methylated DNA, reinforcing gene silencing. This interplay is crucial for maintaining the stability of gene expression programs during development and in response to environmental stimuli.

For example, in stem cells, chromatin accessibility and methylation patterns are highly dynamic, allowing these cells to differentiate into various specialized cell types. In contrast, aberrant coordination of these mechanisms can lead to diseases. In cancer, hypermethylation of promoter regions in tumor suppressor genes often coincides with chromatin compaction, effectively silencing protective pathways.

Clinical Implications

Understanding chromatin accessibility and DNA methylation has transformed biomedical research and clinical practice. These epigenomic markers serve as diagnostic tools and therapeutic targets in various diseases:

Diagnostics: Aberrant methylation patterns are biomarkers for detecting cancers, such as colorectal and lung cancer, even in early stages. Liquid biopsy techniques can identify circulating tumor DNA (ctDNA) with abnormal methylation from a simple blood sample.

The Multi-Omics Revolution

Therapeutics: Epigenetic drugs like DNMT inhibitors (e.g., azacitidine) are used to reverse abnormal DNA methylation in cancers.

Similarly, HDAC inhibitors modulate chromatin accessibility, reactivating silenced genes in malignancies.

Beyond disease, epigenomics has applications in regenerative medicine and aging.

Reprogramming chromatin accessibility and methylation patterns could rejuvenate aged cells or enhance their potential for tissue repair.

Future Perspectives

The study of chromatin accessibility and methylation is rapidly evolving with the advent of single-cell technologies. These methods reveal how epigenomic landscapes differ among individual cells, offering unprecedented insights into developmental biology and disease heterogeneity.

Moreover, integrating epigenomics with other "omics" layers—such as transcriptomics and proteomics—provides a holistic view of cellular regulation.

Epigenomics also holds promise for personalized medicine. By characterizing an individual's unique epigenetic profile, tailored interventions can be developed to restore healthy gene expression patterns.

In conclusion, chromatin accessibility and DNA methylation are fundamental components of the epigenomic landscape, orchestrating the symphony of gene regulation.

Advances in this field continue to illuminate the complexities of life and offer innovative solutions to pressing medical challenges, heralding a new era in precision healthcare.

Proteomics: Quantitative Single-Cell Proteomics

The field of proteomics, dedicated to studying the structure, function, and interactions of proteins within biological systems, has undergone a revolutionary transformation with the advent of single-cell proteomics.

Proteins, the functional workhorses of the cell, are central to virtually all biological processes.

By quantifying proteins at the single-cell level, researchers are uncovering new dimensions of cellular behavior and diversity that were previously obscured by bulk analyses.

Why Single-Cell Proteomics Matters

Traditional proteomics methods analyze large cell populations, producing average measurements that mask heterogeneity among individual cells.

While effective for many applications, bulk approaches cannot resolve cellular variations that play crucial roles in processes like differentiation, immune response, and disease progression.

For example, in cancer, even a small subset of aberrant cells can drive tumor growth and metastasis. Similarly, in neuroscience, cellular heterogeneity underpins the complexity of neural networks.

Quantitative single-cell proteomics enables the measurement of protein expression levels, modifications, and interactions in individual cells.

This approach provides a high-resolution view of cellular states, offering insights into rare cell populations, stochastic gene expression, and dynamic responses to environmental stimuli.

The Technology Behind Single-Cell Proteomics

The Multi-Omics Revolution

Achieving single-cell proteomics is technically challenging due to the small amount of protein present in a single cell.

Several breakthroughs in technology and methodology have made this possible:

Sample Preparation: Techniques like microfluidics and laser-capture microdissection isolate single cells from complex tissues with high precision.

Advanced lysis methods ensure efficient protein extraction from these minute samples.

Protein Identification and Quantification: Mass spectrometry (MS), particularly tandem mass spectrometry (MS/MS), has become the cornerstone of single-cell proteomics.

It enables the identification of thousands of proteins from a single cell by analyzing peptide fragments.

Label-free quantification and isotopic labeling strategies enhance the accuracy of protein quantification.

Sensitivity Enhancements: Innovations such as nanoflow liquid chromatography (nanoLC) and ultra-sensitive mass spectrometers maximize protein detection sensitivity.

Techniques like Single-Cell ProtEomics by Mass Spectrometry (SCoPE-MS) leverage tandem mass tags (TMTs) to multiplex samples, boosting throughput and reducing measurement variability.

Bioinformatics Tools: Advanced algorithms and machine learning models analyze the vast datasets generated, enabling researchers to identify patterns, infer protein functions, and map cellular signaling networks.

Applications of Quantitative Single-Cell Proteomics

Cancer Research: Single-cell proteomics uncovers tumor heterogeneity, identifying subpopulations with distinct proteomic profiles that may resist treatment. It also aids in characterizing the tumor microenvironment, revealing interactions between cancer cells and immune cells.

Immunology: By analyzing immune cells at the single-cell level, researchers can decode immune responses, identify rare cell types like regulatory T cells, and track how immune cells respond to pathogens or vaccines.

Neuroscience: Proteomic studies of neurons and glial cells provide insights into brain function and disorders such as Alzheimer's disease and autism. These studies also shed light on synaptic plasticity and neural circuit formation.

Developmental Biology: Quantitative single-cell proteomics reveals how protein expression changes as cells differentiate into specialized types. This knowledge is critical for understanding developmental processes and regenerative medicine.

Drug Development: Single-cell proteomics accelerates drug discovery by identifying biomarkers for disease states and predicting responses to therapeutic interventions. It also enables the study of drug-target interactions at an unprecedented resolution.

Challenges and Future Directions

Despite its promise, single-cell proteomics faces several challenges:

Sample Loss and Contamination: Handling tiny amounts of protein increases the risk of sample loss and contamination. Improving microfluidic and nanotechnological approaches can mitigate these issues.

The Multi-Omics Revolution

Coverage and Sensitivity: Even with current advancements, detecting low-abundance proteins remains difficult. Further enhancements in mass spectrometry sensitivity and the development of new amplification methods are needed.

Data Complexity: Analyzing single-cell proteomics data requires sophisticated computational tools to handle noise and extract meaningful biological information. Continued development of bioinformatics pipelines is crucial.

Cost and Accessibility: The high cost of instrumentation and reagents limits the widespread adoption of single-cell proteomics. Collaborative efforts to develop cost-effective methods will expand its accessibility.

Looking forward, the integration of single-cell proteomics with other multi-omics technologies promises to deepen our understanding of cellular function. Combining proteomics with single-cell transcriptomics, metabolomics, and epigenomics will provide a more comprehensive picture of cellular biology. For instance, integrating protein and RNA data can reveal how post-transcriptional regulation influences cellular states.

Emerging technologies, such as real-time single-cell proteomics and spatial proteomics, will further enhance the field. Real-time analysis will allow dynamic monitoring of cellular responses, while spatial techniques will map protein distributions within tissues, preserving the context of cellular microenvironments.

Quantitative single-cell proteomics represents a transformative leap in our ability to study biology at the most fundamental level. By capturing the proteomic landscape of individual cells, researchers are uncovering hidden layers of complexity that drive health and disease.

As technologies continue to advance, single-cell proteomics will become an indispensable tool for precision medicine, systems biology, and beyond, ultimately reshaping our understanding of life's molecular machinery.

Metabolomics: Profiling Small Molecules at the Cellular Level

Metabolomics, an integral part of the multi-omics revolution, is the study of small molecules—commonly referred to as metabolites—within cells, tissues, and biological systems. Metabolites are the end products of cellular processes, and their concentrations reflect the dynamic interplay between an organism's genetic blueprint (genome), its protein expression (proteome), and environmental influences. By analyzing these small molecules, metabolomics offers a direct window into the biochemical activities and physiological states of a system, making it a powerful tool in biology and medicine.

What is Metabolomics?

Metabolomics aims to comprehensively profile the metabolome, the complete set of metabolites within a biological sample. These metabolites include sugars, amino acids, lipids, nucleotides, and many other small molecules involved in fundamental biological functions. Unlike genes or proteins, metabolites represent the functional outputs of cellular processes, providing real-time snapshots of the organism's biochemical state.

The field combines advanced analytical techniques, computational tools, and biochemical insights to measure and interpret metabolite levels. It bridges the gap between upstream molecular information (genes and proteins) and downstream physiological outcomes, making it indispensable for understanding complex biological systems.

Key Analytical Techniques in Metabolomics

The success of metabolomics depends heavily on sophisticated technologies that can detect and quantify small molecules with high sensitivity and specificity.

The most commonly used analytical techniques include:

Mass Spectrometry (MS):

MS is a cornerstone of metabolomics, enabling the identification and quantification of metabolites based on their mass-to-charge ratio. Coupled with separation techniques such as gas chromatography (GC) or liquid chromatography (LC), MS can resolve complex mixtures and provide detailed metabolic profiles.

Nuclear Magnetic Resonance (NMR) Spectroscopy:

NMR spectroscopy offers a non-destructive method for analyzing metabolites in solution. While its sensitivity is lower than MS, NMR excels in providing structural information and absolute quantification without the need for prior chemical separation.

Chromatography:

Techniques like gas chromatography and liquid chromatography are often used in conjunction with MS or NMR to separate metabolites based on their physical or chemical properties.

This enhances the resolution and accuracy of metabolite identification.

These tools, combined with bioinformatics and cheminformatics, allow researchers to construct detailed metabolic maps and infer biological pathways.

Applications of Metabolomics

Metabolomics has transformative potential across numerous fields, ranging from medicine and agriculture to environmental science and systems biology.

Healthcare and Precision Medicine:

In medicine, metabolomics is used to identify biomarkers for diseases, enabling earlier diagnoses and personalized treatment plans.

For example, metabolic signatures can reveal insights into cancer, diabetes, cardiovascular diseases, and neurological disorders. Metabolomics also supports drug discovery by elucidating drug metabolism and potential side effects.

Nutritional Science:

Metabolomics provides insights into how diet and nutrition influence metabolic pathways. It can assess how different foods affect an individual's metabolism and identify optimal dietary interventions for health and disease prevention.

Agriculture and Crop Science:

In agriculture, metabolomics is applied to improve crop yield, resistance to pests, and stress tolerance. By understanding plant metabolomes, researchers can engineer crops with enhanced nutritional profiles and resilience to environmental challenges.

Environmental Science:

Metabolomics helps monitor the impact of pollutants on ecosystems by profiling metabolic changes in organisms exposed to environmental stressors. This application is crucial for assessing the health of ecosystems and informing conservation efforts.

Systems Biology and Drug Discovery:

As part of the systems biology toolkit, metabolomics enables the integration of multi-omics data to understand complex biological networks. In drug discovery, it aids in uncovering drug targets and understanding mechanisms of action.

The Multi-Omics Revolution

Challenges in Metabolomics

Despite its immense potential, metabolomics faces several challenges:

Complexity of the Metabolome:

The metabolome is highly dynamic and influenced by numerous factors, including age, diet, microbiome composition, and environmental conditions.

This variability complicates the task of obtaining consistent and reproducible data.

Analytical Limitations:

No single analytical platform can capture the entirety of the metabolome. Combining multiple techniques increases cost and complexity, presenting logistical challenges.

Data Analysis and Interpretation:

The sheer volume of data generated by metabolomic studies necessitates robust computational tools and databases. Extracting meaningful biological insights from this data requires interdisciplinary expertise in biochemistry, statistics, and informatics.

The Future of Metabolomics

The field of metabolomics is evolving rapidly, driven by advances in technology and data science. High-throughput platforms, machine learning algorithms, and improved metabolite databases are enhancing the speed and accuracy of metabolomic analyses.

Integration with other omics disciplines, such as genomics, transcriptomics, and proteomics, is unlocking new dimensions of biological understanding.

For example, by combining metabolomics with microbiomics, researchers are unraveling the intricate relationships between the human gut microbiome and systemic health.

Similarly, the integration of metabolomics with proteomics is shedding light on how enzyme activities regulate metabolic pathways in health and disease.

Metabolomics is a cornerstone of the multi-omics revolution, offering unparalleled insights into cellular processes at the molecular level.

By profiling the small molecules that drive life, it provides a deeper understanding of biology and transforms how we approach health, agriculture, and environmental sustainability.

As technologies improve and interdisciplinary collaborations expand, metabolomics will continue to unlock new frontiers in science and innovation.

This field not only enhances our knowledge of life's complexity but also equips us to address some of the most pressing challenges facing humanity today.

6. Methodologies for Multi-Omics Data Acquisition

Experimental Designs Combining Different Omics Layers

The advent of multi-omics has revolutionized biological research by enabling scientists to investigate complex biological systems in a holistic manner. Multi-omics integrates various omics layers, such as genomics, transcriptomics, proteomics, metabolomics, and epigenomics, to provide a comprehensive view of biological processes. Designing experiments that effectively combine these omics layers requires strategic planning to ensure meaningful integration, robust data acquisition, and insightful interpretation.

This page delves into the principles, methodologies, and challenges associated with experimental designs in multi-omics research.

The Rationale for Integrating Omics Layers

Biological systems are intricate and operate at multiple molecular levels.

Each omics layer provides unique insights into specific aspects of these systems:

Genomics reveals the static blueprint of an organism, detailing the DNA sequence and structural variations.

Transcriptomics highlights the dynamic expression of genes, offering insights into cellular responses to various stimuli.

Proteomics uncovers the functional molecules of the cell, shedding light on protein interactions, modifications, and activity.

Metabolomics provides a snapshot of the biochemical activities within cells by profiling small molecules and metabolites.

Epigenomics investigates modifications to the DNA and chromatin structure that regulate gene expression without altering the sequence.

By combining these layers, researchers can uncover connections between genotype and phenotype, elucidate disease mechanisms, and identify biomarkers or therapeutic targets.

Key Principles of Multi-Omics Experimental Design

Define Clear Objectives

The research question drives the experimental design. Clear objectives ensure that the integration of omics layers aligns with the study's goals. For example, investigating cancer progression might require genomics and transcriptomics to identify mutations and expression changes, coupled with metabolomics to understand altered metabolic pathways.

Select Appropriate Omics Layers

Not all omics layers are necessary for every study. The choice depends on the biological question. Integrating fewer but relevant layers often yields more focused and actionable insights.

Harmonize Sample Collection and Processing

Consistent sample collection and processing protocols are critical to minimize variability. Ideally, all omics data should originate from the same biological sample to maintain coherence.

Prioritize Data Quality and Compatibility

High-quality data acquisition from each omics layer is essential. Technologies and platforms should be chosen for their sensitivity, reproducibility, and compatibility with downstream analyses.

Design for Computational Integration

Integration relies on advanced computational tools and statistical methods.

Ensuring datasets are compatible in terms of scale, resolution, and format simplifies the integration process.

Strategies for Combining Omics Layers

Sequential Omics Analysis

In this approach, data from one omics layer informs the choice of subsequent layers.

For example, transcriptomic data might identify key genes of interest, which are then investigated at the proteomic or metabolomic levels.

Parallel Omics Analysis

All omics layers are analyzed simultaneously, providing a comprehensive view of the system. This approach demands meticulous planning to ensure synchronization across platforms and analytical workflows.

Time-Series Multi-Omics

Observing dynamic changes over time by collecting multi-omics data at different time points is particularly useful in understanding developmental processes or disease progression.

Spatial Multi-Omics

Spatially resolved omics integrates molecular data with spatial information, revealing how cellular environments and locations influence molecular interactions.

Techniques like spatial transcriptomics or imaging mass spectrometry are increasingly applied in this context.

Challenges in Multi-Omics Experimental Design

Technical and Analytical Complexity

Combining omics layers involves handling diverse technologies, each with unique requirements and limitations.

For instance, genomics often involves high-throughput sequencing, while proteomics relies on mass spectrometry.

Data Integration and Interpretation

Integrating large, heterogeneous datasets is computationally intensive. Different data types may vary in scale (e.g., transcript counts versus metabolite concentrations), requiring sophisticated normalization and modeling techniques.

Cost and Resource Constraints

Multi-omics studies are resource-intensive, often requiring significant financial investment and access to specialized equipment and expertise.

Reproducibility and Validation

Ensuring reproducibility across omics layers is challenging due to variability in data acquisition and analysis methods.

Rigorous validation of findings is critical.

The Multi-Omics Revolution

Applications and Case Studies

Multi-omics approaches have been transformative in various fields:

Cancer Research: Integrating genomics, transcriptomics, and proteomics has enabled the identification of oncogenic pathways and personalized therapeutic targets.

Microbiome Studies: Combining metagenomics with metabolomics reveals the functional impact of microbial communities on host health.

Plant Biology: Multi-omics approaches unravel the genetic and metabolic networks underlying stress responses, aiding crop improvement efforts.

One notable case involves the study of Alzheimer's disease, where researchers combined transcriptomics, proteomics, and metabolomics to identify biomarkers and pathways associated with disease onset.

This comprehensive approach has provided a deeper understanding of disease mechanisms, paving the way for novel diagnostic and therapeutic strategies.

Future Directions

As technologies advance, multi-omics experimental designs are poised to become even more powerful. Emerging trends include:

Single-Cell Multi-Omics: Integrating omics layers at the single-cell level provides unprecedented resolution, enabling the study of cellular heterogeneity.

AI and Machine Learning: These tools are revolutionizing data integration, pattern recognition, and predictive modeling in multi-omics research.

Global Collaborations: Sharing datasets and expertise across institutions accelerates discoveries and enhances reproducibility.

By embracing these advancements, scientists can unlock deeper insights into the complexities of life, driving innovations in medicine, agriculture, and beyond.

The multi-omics revolution is not just about combining data; it is about transforming our understanding of biology.

Barcoding and Spatial Techniques

The field of multi-omics has transformed our understanding of biological systems, enabling scientists to investigate the intricate interplay of molecules within cells, tissues, and organisms. Among the cutting-edge technologies driving this revolution are barcoding and spatial techniques.

These tools provide unparalleled insights into cellular heterogeneity, spatial organization, and the dynamics of molecular interactions, bridging the gap between molecular biology and spatial context.

Barcoding Techniques: Decoding Cellular Complexity

Barcoding techniques are innovative methods used to tag and identify individual cells, molecules, or genomic fragments within a biological sample.

By assigning unique molecular "barcodes" to specific entities, researchers can track their origins, interactions, and behaviors across complex datasets.

These techniques are pivotal for high-throughput studies such as single-cell omics, enabling the analysis of thousands or even millions of individual cells in a single experiment.

The Multi-Omics Revolution

How Barcoding Works

At its core, barcoding involves attaching a unique sequence of nucleotides to molecules of interest. This sequence serves as a molecular identifier, much like a grocery store barcode.

For instance, in single-cell RNA sequencing (scRNA-seq), barcodes are added to RNA molecules extracted from individual cells.

After sequencing, the barcodes enable researchers to assign reads back to their respective cells, creating a detailed map of gene expression at the single-cell level.

Applications of Barcoding

Single-Cell Analysis: Barcoding allows scientists to explore cellular diversity, identify rare cell populations, and uncover novel cell types. This has profound implications for understanding development, disease progression, and immune responses.

Lineage Tracing: Barcodes can be introduced into cells at specific time points to track their lineage and differentiation over time.

This is especially useful in developmental biology and cancer research.

High-Throughput Screening: By tagging individual genetic variants or drug candidates with barcodes, researchers can assess their effects in parallel, streamlining drug discovery and functional genomics.

Barcoding has democratized access to high-resolution biological data, but it is not without challenges. Ensuring accuracy in barcode assignment, managing sequencing errors, and analyzing massive datasets require sophisticated computational tools and algorithms.

Spatial Techniques: Mapping Biology in 3D

While barcoding excels at unraveling molecular diversity, spatial techniques add another critical layer of understanding by preserving and analyzing the spatial organization of biological molecules within tissues.

These techniques capture the "where" of molecular activity, offering insights into how cellular and molecular interactions are influenced by their physical environment.

Principles of Spatial Techniques

Spatial omics combines molecular profiling with spatially resolved imaging, retaining the architecture of the tissue or organ being studied.

Unlike traditional bulk analysis, where spatial context is lost, these techniques enable researchers to observe how cells and molecules are distributed and interact in their native environments.

Key spatial omics approaches include:

Spatial Transcriptomics: This technique maps RNA expression across tissue sections, linking gene expression profiles to specific locations within the tissue.

Advances in this field have led to the development of platforms like 10x Genomics Visium and NanoString GeoMx.

Spatial Proteomics: By analyzing protein distributions, researchers can investigate cellular signaling pathways, immune responses, and disease mechanisms with high spatial resolution.

Spatial Metabolomics: Mapping metabolite distributions provides insights into metabolic heterogeneity and microenvironmental influences, such as those seen in tumor biology.

Applications of Spatial Techniques

Tumor Microenvironment: Spatial omics reveals how cancer cells interact with their surrounding stromal and immune cells, shedding light on mechanisms of tumor growth and resistance.

Neuroscience: By mapping gene and protein expression in brain tissues, spatial techniques uncover the molecular underpinnings of brain function and neurological disorders.

Developmental Biology: These methods visualize cellular differentiation and tissue organization during embryonic development.

Integrating Barcoding and Spatial Techniques

The combination of barcoding and spatial techniques represents a powerful synergy in multi-omics research.

Together, they provide a comprehensive view of biological systems, capturing both the molecular diversity and the spatial context in which these molecules operate.

For example, spatial transcriptomics data can be enriched with single-cell RNA-seq barcoding to validate findings and identify cell-type-specific signatures within tissues.

One exciting application is in the study of immune responses.

Barcoding enables the identification of diverse immune cell populations, while spatial techniques reveal how these cells are organized within tissues during infection or inflammation.

This integrated approach offers a holistic view of the immune system in action.

Future Directions and Challenges

As these technologies advance, their potential continues to expand. Researchers are developing hybrid platforms that combine barcoding and spatial techniques in a single workflow, enhancing data integration and reducing experimental complexity. AI and machine learning are also playing a crucial role in processing and interpreting the massive datasets generated by these methods.

However, challenges remain. The high cost of instrumentation and consumables limits accessibility, and data integration across different omics layers requires sophisticated computational frameworks.

Additionally, maintaining sample integrity and resolving molecular signals in dense tissues are ongoing technical hurdles.

Barcoding and spatial techniques are revolutionizing our ability to study biological systems with unprecedented detail. By dissecting molecular diversity and spatial organization, these technologies are driving discoveries in cancer research, immunology, neuroscience, and beyond.

As innovations continue to refine these methods, they hold the promise of unlocking deeper insights into the complex tapestry of life.

The multi-omics revolution is not just a leap forward in technology—it is a profound transformation in how we understand and explore the biology of living systems.

7. Data Integration and Computational Tools

Algorithms for Cross-Omics Integration

The integration of diverse omics data—such as genomics, transcriptomics, proteomics, metabolomics, and epigenomics—has revolutionized the way we understand complex biological systems. These data types capture different layers of biological information, and their integration is key to uncovering comprehensive insights into health, disease, and biological function.

At the heart of this integration lie sophisticated algorithms designed to harmonize, process, and analyze these varied datasets.

The Need for Cross-Omics Integration

Single-omics approaches often fall short in providing a complete picture of biological phenomena.

For instance, genomic data can reveal predispositions to diseases, but combining it with transcriptomics data highlights gene expression patterns, while proteomics and metabolomics provide insights into functional outcomes.

The integration of these datasets requires algorithms capable of managing their inherent differences, including scale, format, noise levels, and missing values.

Types of Algorithms for Cross-Omics Integration

Algorithms for cross-omics integration can be broadly classified into three categories: unsupervised, supervised, and hybrid approaches.

Unsupervised Methods Unsupervised methods focus on uncovering patterns and relationships within multi-omics data without prior knowledge or labeled outcomes.

Common techniques include:

Principal Component Analysis (PCA): PCA reduces the dimensionality of datasets while preserving the most informative features.

By applying it to multiple omics layers, researchers can identify shared components and correlated features across datasets.

Clustering Algorithms: Algorithms like k-means clustering and hierarchical clustering group similar data points across omics layers, helping to identify subtypes of diseases or biological states.

Network-Based Approaches: Methods such as weighted gene co-expression network analysis (WGCNA) build networks to link related features from different omics datasets, offering a graphical representation of interconnected biological processes.

Supervised Methods Supervised methods rely on labeled data to predict outcomes or classify samples.

These algorithms are particularly useful for clinical applications, such as biomarker discovery and disease classification.

Examples include:

Machine Learning Models: Algorithms like support vector machines (SVMs), random forests, and gradient boosting classifiers integrate omics data to predict phenotypes or clinical outcomes.

The Multi-Omics Revolution

Deep Learning: Neural networks, particularly those designed for multi-modal data (e.g., convolutional neural networks and autoencoders), excel in capturing complex relationships across omics layers.

Hybrid Methods Hybrid methods combine the strengths of both supervised and unsupervised approaches.

They often use unsupervised learning to reduce dimensionality or extract features before applying supervised models.

Examples include:

Integration Frameworks: Multi-omics integration frameworks like iCluster and MOFA (Multi-Omics Factor Analysis) are designed to jointly analyze multiple datasets while addressing their heterogeneity.

Bayesian Networks: These probabilistic models integrate omics data by defining dependencies between variables and enabling inference of causal relationships.

Integration Strategies

Effective cross-omics integration requires selecting the appropriate strategy, often determined by the nature of the data and research objectives.

Common strategies include:

Horizontal Integration: This approach combines datasets of the same omics type from different sources or conditions, enhancing the depth of analysis.

Vertical Integration: Vertical integration aligns different omics types (e.g., genomics with proteomics) to create a comprehensive, multi-layered view of biological systems.

Diagonal Integration: A more complex approach that combines elements of both horizontal and vertical integration, enabling the study of cross-talk between similar and distinct omics layers.

Challenges in Algorithm Development

Developing robust algorithms for cross-omics integration is challenging due to several factors:

Data Heterogeneity: Omics datasets vary in scale, format, and underlying biological meaning, making harmonization difficult. Missing Data: Incomplete datasets are common in multi-omics studies, necessitating imputation techniques or algorithms that can handle sparse data.

High Dimensionality: Multi-omics datasets often contain thousands of variables but relatively few samples, increasing the risk of overfitting.

Computational Complexity: Integrating multiple large-scale datasets requires efficient algorithms capable of handling high computational demands.

Applications in Multi-Omics Research

Cross-omics integration has led to breakthroughs across various domains:

Precision Medicine: By integrating patient-specific omics data, algorithms identify personalized treatment options and predict responses to therapy.

Biomarker Discovery: Integrated data analysis uncovers biomarkers with higher predictive power by combining molecular layers.

Systems Biology: Cross-omics approaches map complex biological pathways and uncover interactions between genes, proteins, and metabolites.

The Multi-Omics Revolution

Agrigenomics: In agricultural sciences, cross-omics integration helps improve crop yields and resilience by linking genetic information to phenotypic traits.

Future Directions

Advancements in computational power, algorithm design, and data acquisition technologies promise to further enhance cross-omics integration.

Emerging trends include the development of:

Graph-Based Methods: Algorithms leveraging graph theory for more intuitive and flexible data representation.

Federated Learning: Approaches that enable collaborative multi-omics research across institutions while preserving data privacy.

Explainable AI: Methods that prioritize interpretability, ensuring that insights from integrated analyses are accessible to researchers and clinicians.

In conclusion, algorithms for cross-omics integration are indispensable tools for decoding the complexities of biology.

As these methods continue to evolve, they hold the potential to transform multi-omics research, paving the way for innovations in science and medicine.

Visualization and Interpretation of Multi-Dimensional Data

The ever-growing volume of data generated through multi-omics technologies has revolutionized our understanding of biology. However, this progress comes with its own set of challenges, particularly in visualizing and interpreting multi-dimensional data. Multi-omics studies often integrate diverse data types—genomics, transcriptomics, proteomics, epigenomics, and metabolomics—each providing unique insights into biological systems. Understanding how to effectively visualize and interpret this information is critical for uncovering hidden patterns, drawing meaningful conclusions, and translating findings into actionable knowledge.

The Complexity of Multi-Omics Data

Multi-omics datasets are inherently multi-dimensional, with each omics layer contributing thousands or even millions of variables. For example, a transcriptomics dataset may include the expression levels of thousands of genes, while a proteomics dataset might capture a vast array of protein interactions and concentrations. These data types are often heterogeneous, non-linear, and influenced by numerous confounding factors. Thus, visualizing this data requires tools that can handle complexity without overwhelming researchers.

The Role of Visualization in Multi-Omics

Visualization transforms raw, complex data into interpretable and intuitive formats, enabling researchers to identify patterns, relationships, and anomalies. Effective visualization tools must balance simplicity and depth, providing a clear overview while allowing exploration of finer details.

From uncovering gene-disease associations to identifying biomarkers and predicting therapeutic targets, visualization plays a pivotal role in all stages of multi-omics research.

Common Visualization Techniques

The Multi-Omics Revolution

A variety of visualization techniques have been developed for multi-omics data.

Here are some of the most commonly used approaches:

Heatmaps: Heatmaps are widely used to display the relationships between variables. For instance, in transcriptomics studies, heatmaps can show gene expression levels across multiple samples.

Clustering algorithms often complement heatmaps, grouping similar data points to reveal patterns.

Principal Component Analysis (PCA): PCA is a dimensionality reduction technique that simplifies multi-dimensional data by projecting it onto fewer dimensions.

The reduced dimensions are visualized as scatterplots, making it easier to identify clusters or outliers.

Network Graphs: Biological systems are inherently interconnected, and network graphs excel at representing relationships between entities such as genes, proteins, or metabolites.

These graphs can highlight key hubs and pathways central to specific biological processes.

Circos Plots: Circos plots are circular representations often used to illustrate genomic variations, such as structural rearrangements, or to map interactions between different omics layers.

They are particularly useful for displaying relationships across multiple datasets in a visually engaging manner.

Sankey Diagrams: These flow diagrams are ideal for tracking the integration and movement of information between different omics layers, such as gene expression influencing protein abundance and metabolite production.

T-distributed Stochastic Neighbor Embedding (t-SNE) and Uniform Manifold Approximation and Projection (UMAP):

These non-linear dimensionality reduction methods are particularly effective for visualizing high-dimensional data, enabling researchers to detect subtle patterns and relationships in a 2D or 3D space.

Interpretation Challenges

Interpreting multi-omics data requires careful consideration of the context in which the data was generated.

Some challenges include:

Data Integration: Combining different omics layers often introduces biases and noise.

Visualization tools must account for these factors to provide accurate interpretations.

Biological Relevance: Not all observed patterns are biologically meaningful.

Statistical analyses and domain expertise are critical for distinguishing significant findings from noise.

Scalability: As datasets grow larger, traditional visualization methods may struggle to handle the volume of data.

Scalable visualization techniques that retain clarity are essential.

The Multi-Omics Revolution

Emerging Tools and Technologies

Recent advances in computational tools have significantly improved the visualization and interpretation of multi-omics data.

Machine learning and artificial intelligence are playing a transformative role by uncovering complex relationships that traditional methods might miss.

Platforms like Cytoscape, OmicsNet, and iDEP are equipped with user-friendly interfaces, enabling researchers to create complex visualizations without extensive coding knowledge.

Interactive visualization tools are also gaining traction. For example, Shiny apps in R and Plotly in Python allow dynamic exploration of datasets, enabling users to zoom in on specific data points, adjust parameters, and view results in real time.

These tools empower researchers to interact with data, fostering deeper insights.

The Human Factor in Visualization

Beyond technical challenges, effective visualization must prioritize human usability.

Clarity, simplicity, and intuitive design are essential to ensure that visualizations communicate findings effectively.

Color schemes, labeling, and layout design should cater to diverse audiences, from computational biologists to clinicians.

Employing storytelling principles in visualization can further enhance interpretability, guiding viewers through the narrative of the data.

Bridging the Gap Between Data and Discovery

Visualization and interpretation are not just tools for understanding; they are bridges connecting data to actionable discovery.

By integrating intuitive visualizations with robust statistical frameworks, researchers can turn multi-dimensional data into breakthroughs in medicine, agriculture, environmental science, and beyond.

In conclusion, mastering the visualization and interpretation of multi-dimensional data is essential for harnessing the full potential of the multi-omics revolution.

As computational tools continue to evolve, researchers are increasingly equipped to tackle the challenges of complexity, paving the way for deeper insights and transformative discoveries.

8. Standardization and Quality Control

Ensuring Reproducibility in Multi-Omics Studies

Reproducibility is a cornerstone of scientific research, ensuring that findings are reliable and applicable across different settings and studies. In multi-omics research, where data is collected from diverse biological layers—such as genomics, transcriptomics, proteomics, metabolomics, and epigenomics—reproducibility becomes even more crucial yet challenging. This complexity arises from the sheer volume of data, varying experimental conditions, and intricate computational analyses required.

Here, we delve into the key strategies and considerations for ensuring reproducibility in multi-omics studies in a manner that is accessible and practical.

Standardization of Experimental Protocols
One of the first steps toward reproducibility is the standardization of experimental protocols. Variations in sample collection, preparation, and storage can introduce biases, making it difficult to replicate findings. For instance, the timing of sample collection, environmental conditions, or even subtle differences in reagent batches can impact results. Establishing and following well-documented, standardized protocols ensures consistency.

Moreover, sharing these protocols openly with the research community promotes transparency and allows others to replicate the methodologies accurately.

Quality Control and Validation

Ensuring high-quality data is fundamental to reproducibility. Quality control (QC) measures should be applied at every stage, from sample acquisition to data analysis. Techniques such as spectrophotometric analysis to verify sample purity, benchmarking computational tools, and cross-validation using independent datasets are essential steps. Employing biological and technical replicates further strengthens the reliability of results by accounting for natural variability and potential experimental errors.

Validation of findings through independent datasets or alternative methods provides additional assurance. For example, results derived from transcriptomics can be corroborated using proteomics data, offering a multi-layered perspective that enhances reliability.

Comprehensive Metadata Documentation

Metadata—information about the data—plays a critical role in ensuring reproducibility. Comprehensive metadata includes details about sample collection, experimental conditions, instrument settings, and data processing workflows. Accurate and thorough documentation helps researchers understand the context of the data, making it easier to replicate the study. Initiatives such as the Minimum Information About a Microarray Experiment (MIAME) guidelines have set a benchmark for metadata reporting, and similar frameworks are emerging for multi-omics studies.

Robust Computational Pipelines

In multi-omics research, the computational analysis is as significant as the experimental work. The choice of software, algorithms, and statistical methods can greatly influence results. Employing robust and well-documented computational pipelines is essential for reproducibility. Open-source tools and platforms, which allow other researchers to examine and reuse the code, are highly encouraged.

The Multi-Omics Revolution

Version control systems such as GitHub and containerization tools like Docker or Singularity can further enhance reproducibility by ensuring consistent computational environments.

These tools help researchers track changes in analysis workflows and recreate the exact conditions under which the original analysis was performed.

Addressing Batch Effects

Batch effects, or systematic differences between groups of samples processed at different times or under varying conditions, are a common challenge in multi-omics studies. If unaddressed, these effects can lead to false conclusions. Statistical methods such as ComBat or surrogate variable analysis (SVA) are widely used to correct batch effects.

Additionally, designing experiments to minimize batch variability—by randomizing sample processing orders or including controls across batches—can prevent these issues from arising.

Open Data Sharing

Open data sharing is a powerful approach to enhancing reproducibility. By making raw and processed data publicly accessible through repositories such as Gene Expression Omnibus (GEO), Proteomics Identifications Database (PRIDE), or MetaboLights, researchers allow others to validate and build upon their findings. Open data also fosters collaboration and accelerates scientific discovery.

However, open data sharing must be accompanied by adherence to data privacy regulations, especially in studies involving human participants. Ethical considerations and proper de-identification of sensitive data are paramount to maintaining trust and compliance.

Rigorous Statistical Analysis

The statistical methods used in multi-omics studies must be carefully chosen to account for the complexity of the data. High-dimensional data and the integration of multiple omics layers pose unique statistical challenges, such as the risk of overfitting or false positives.

Techniques like cross-validation, permutation testing, and multi-layer data integration frameworks help mitigate these risks. Clear reporting of statistical methodologies, including the rationale behind their selection, is critical for reproducibility.

Cross-Study Validation

Reproducibility is ultimately demonstrated when findings are validated across independent studies. Cross-study validation involves applying a study's findings or computational models to external datasets.

This practice not only confirms the robustness of the original results but also reveals potential limitations or context-specific factors influencing the outcomes.

Education and Training

Promoting a culture of reproducibility requires ongoing education and training. Researchers must be equipped with the knowledge and tools to design reproducible studies, handle complex multi-omics datasets, and perform rigorous analyses.

Workshops, online courses, and collaborative networks can help build these competencies within the scientific community.

Ensuring reproducibility in multi-omics studies is a multifaceted endeavor that requires careful planning, transparent practices, and collaborative efforts.

By standardizing protocols, maintaining high data quality, employing robust computational tools, and embracing open science principles, researchers can overcome the challenges inherent in this field.

As multi-omics continues to revolutionize our understanding of biology and disease, prioritizing reproducibility will ensure that its findings are not only groundbreaking but also trustworthy and impactful for years to come.

Data Normalization Across Omics Layers

The emergence of multi-omics approaches—integrating genomics, transcriptomics, proteomics, metabolomics, and epigenomics—has revolutionized our ability to investigate biological systems at unprecedented depth. However, the complexity and variability inherent to each omics layer pose a significant challenge to achieving accurate, meaningful, and integrative insights.

One of the most critical steps in multi-omics analysis is data normalization, which ensures that data from different omics layers can be effectively compared and analyzed in a cohesive manner.

This process is essential to remove biases, reduce technical noise, and allow biological signals to shine through.

Understanding the Need for Data Normalization

Data generated from different omics platforms are highly diverse in nature.

For instance:

Genomic data often comprises binary or categorical variables representing the presence or absence of mutations.

Transcriptomic data involves continuous measurements of RNA expression levels, typically quantified as raw read counts or fragments per kilobase of transcript per million mapped reads (FPKM).

Proteomic data measures protein abundances, which can vary significantly depending on experimental protocols and instrumentation.

Metabolomic data spans a wide range of molecular concentrations, from picomolar to millimolar, making it particularly prone to scale disparities.

These variations arise not only from biological differences but also from technical factors such as sequencing depth, sample preparation methods, and instrument sensitivity.

Without normalization, downstream analyses risk being skewed by these technical artifacts, leading to erroneous conclusions.

Key Challenges in Multi-Omics Data Normalization

Heterogeneous Data Types: Each omics layer generates data of varying formats, distributions, and scales. For example, RNA-seq data often follows a negative binomial distribution, while proteomic data may exhibit log-normal characteristics.

Batch Effects: Samples processed in different batches can show significant variation due to differences in reagents, equipment, or operator handling.

Missing Values: Omics datasets frequently contain missing values, especially in proteomics and metabolomics, due to limitations in detection sensitivity.

Biological and Technical Noise: Disentangling true biological variation from noise introduced during sample collection and processing is a complex task.

The Multi-Omics Revolution

Integration Across Scales: Combining omics datasets requires normalization methods that account for scale differences while preserving meaningful biological relationships.

Methods for Data Normalization

Various normalization techniques have been developed to address these challenges. The choice of method depends on the specific omics layer and the nature of the dataset.

1. Scaling and Transformation

Log Transformation: Converts data to a log scale to reduce skewness and make distributions more symmetric.

Z-Score Normalization: Centers data by subtracting the mean and scales it by dividing by the standard deviation, making datasets comparable.

Quantile Normalization: Ensures that the distributions of data from different samples are identical.

2. Batch Effect Correction

ComBat: A widely used method for correcting batch effects by using empirical Bayes frameworks.

Surrogate Variable Analysis (SVA): Identifies hidden factors causing variability and adjusts for them.

3. Count-Based Normalization (For Transcriptomics)

TPM (Transcripts Per Million): Normalizes RNA-seq data by accounting for gene length and sequencing depth.

DESeq2 and EdgeR: Use sophisticated statistical models to normalize count data for differential expression analysis.

4. Missing Data Imputation

Machine learning methods like k-nearest neighbors (k-NN) or matrix factorization are commonly applied to impute missing values.

5. Multi-Omics-Specific Normalization

Cross-Platform Normalization: Algorithms such as Multiple Factor Analysis (MFA) or Multi-Omics Factor Analysis (MOFA) allow normalization across omics layers while retaining inter-omics relationships.

Workflow for Effective Data Normalization

A systematic workflow is essential for successful data normalization:

Data Preprocessing: Begin by removing outliers and performing quality checks to ensure reliable data input.

Layer-Specific Normalization: Apply normalization techniques tailored to the characteristics of each omics layer.

Batch Effect Correction: Use tools like ComBat to eliminate inter-batch variability.

Integration Preparation: Employ methods such as scaling or feature matching to align datasets from different omics layers.

Validation: Verify that the biological signals of interest are preserved after normalization.

The Multi-Omics Revolution

Advances and Future Directions

Recent advances in machine learning and artificial intelligence have opened new avenues for data normalization. Deep learning models, such as autoencoders, can learn complex patterns in multi-omics data, enabling more nuanced normalization and integration.

Additionally, federated learning approaches allow collaborative normalization across institutions while preserving data privacy.

Moreover, the development of benchmarking frameworks, such as the OpenOmics platform, provides researchers with tools to evaluate the performance of normalization methods.

These innovations are expected to enhance the reproducibility and robustness of multi-omics studies.

Data normalization across omics layers is a cornerstone of multi-omics research, enabling the integration of diverse datasets into a unified framework.

By addressing the inherent variability in multi-omics data, normalization allows researchers to uncover meaningful biological insights, drive innovation in precision medicine, and unravel the complexities of human health and disease.

As computational tools and statistical methods continue to evolve, the ability to normalize and integrate multi-omics data will become increasingly sophisticated, paving the way for transformative discoveries.

9. Developmental Biology

Insights into Cell Differentiation and Lineage Tracing

Developmental biology is a cornerstone of understanding how complex organisms arise from a single cell. This intricate journey, guided by genetic instructions and influenced by environmental cues, unfolds through the processes of cell differentiation and lineage tracing.

Recent advances in multi-omics technologies are revolutionizing our ability to explore these phenomena, providing unprecedented insights into the molecular and cellular orchestration that drives development.

The Fundamentals of Cell Differentiation

Cell differentiation is the process by which unspecialized progenitor cells develop into distinct cell types with specialized functions. This transformation is fundamental to the creation of tissues and organs during embryogenesis and is driven by tightly regulated changes in gene expression.

Key mechanisms underlying differentiation include:

Epigenetic Modifications: DNA methylation, histone modifications, and chromatin remodeling dictate the accessibility of genes, turning them "on" or "off" in response to developmental cues.

Transcriptional Regulation: Specific transcription factors bind to DNA sequences to activate or repress genes essential for cell fate decisions.

The Multi-Omics Revolution

Signal Transduction Pathways: Extracellular signals, such as growth factors, activate intracellular pathways that steer differentiation by modulating gene expression and cellular behavior.

These mechanisms work in concert to ensure that the right cells emerge at the right time and place, creating the diversity of cell types required for a functional organism.

The Role of Lineage Tracing in Developmental Biology

Understanding how individual cells give rise to specific cell types and tissues is central to developmental biology. Lineage tracing is a technique used to map the progeny of a single cell over time, shedding light on the dynamics of development and tissue regeneration.

Traditional lineage tracing methods relied on markers like dyes or genetic reporters, but these approaches were limited in resolution and scope.

Modern advancements have introduced fate-mapping techniques, such as:

Genetic Barcoding: Unique DNA sequences are introduced into cells, acting as identifiers to trace their descendants.

Single-Cell Multi-Omics: By integrating genomics, transcriptomics, and epigenomics at the single-cell level, researchers can reconstruct lineage relationships with remarkable precision.

CRISPR-Cas9-based Approaches: This technology enables the introduction of unique mutations or tags in specific cells, allowing for high-resolution lineage mapping.

These innovations have transformed lineage tracing into a powerful tool for unraveling the complexities of development and regeneration.

Multi-Omics: A Game-Changer in Developmental Biology

The integration of multi-omics technologies—spanning genomics, transcriptomics, proteomics, metabolomics, and epigenomics—has unlocked new dimensions of understanding in developmental biology. By capturing the interplay between various molecular layers, multi-omics provides a holistic view of cell differentiation and lineage specification.

Single-Cell Transcriptomics:

High-throughput sequencing of RNA from individual cells reveals dynamic gene expression changes during differentiation. It enables the identification of rare cell types and transitional states that were previously elusive.

Epigenomics:

Techniques like ATAC-seq and ChIP-seq uncover epigenetic landscapes that regulate gene accessibility.

These insights are critical for understanding how stem cells commit to specific lineages.

Proteomics and Metabolomics:

Proteomics elucidates protein expression and modifications, providing functional insights into cell states.

Metabolomics tracks metabolic shifts that support the energy demands of differentiation.

Spatial Omics:

Emerging technologies like spatial transcriptomics retain the spatial context of cells, allowing researchers to map gene expression within tissues.

The Multi-Omics Revolution

By integrating these data layers, multi-omics paints a comprehensive picture of how cells transition through various developmental stages, bridging gaps in our understanding of the molecular drivers of differentiation.

Applications and Implications

The insights gained from multi-omics studies have profound implications for both basic and applied sciences.

Key applications include:

Regenerative Medicine: Understanding differentiation pathways informs strategies to generate specific cell types for therapeutic purposes, such as replacing damaged neurons or regenerating heart tissue.

Cancer Research: Many cancers arise from disruptions in differentiation. Multi-omics helps decipher how these processes go awry, guiding the development of targeted therapies.

Evolutionary Biology: Comparing differentiation mechanisms across species illuminates how developmental processes have evolved to produce diverse forms of life.

Challenges and Future Directions
Despite its transformative potential, multi-omics research faces several challenges:

Data Integration: Combining and interpreting diverse datasets from different omics layers requires advanced computational tools and expertise.

Cost and Accessibility: High-throughput technologies can be expensive, limiting their widespread adoption.

Dynamic Processes: Developmental processes are highly dynamic, necessitating time-resolved multi-omics approaches to capture changes in real-time.

Future efforts aim to refine multi-omics methodologies, enhance data interpretation through machine learning, and expand their accessibility to broader research communities.

By doing so, we can further decode the mysteries of development and harness this knowledge for innovative applications.

Cell differentiation and lineage tracing lie at the heart of developmental biology, shaping the way we understand life's blueprint.

The multi-omics revolution has opened new frontiers in this field, providing detailed, system-wide insights into the molecular mechanisms that drive these processes.

As technologies continue to evolve, the promise of unlocking the full potential of developmental biology grows ever closer, paving the way for breakthroughs in medicine, biotechnology, and beyond.

10. Cancer Research

Tumor Heterogeneity and Clonal Evolution

Tumor heterogeneity and clonal evolution are central themes in modern cancer biology, reshaping our understanding of how cancers develop, evolve, and respond to treatment.

With the advent of multi-omics approaches, scientists are unraveling the complex interplay of genetic, epigenetic, transcriptomic, proteomic, and metabolomic factors that drive tumor behavior.

This holistic perspective is transforming our ability to diagnose, monitor, and treat cancers more effectively.

Tumor Heterogeneity: A Complex Landscape

Tumor heterogeneity refers to the diversity observed within and between tumors at multiple levels. Two main types of heterogeneity exist: inter-tumor heterogeneity, which represents differences between tumors in different patients, and intra-tumor heterogeneity, describing variations within a single tumor.

Genetic Heterogeneity

Genetic diversity arises from mutations, chromosomal rearrangements, and copy number variations. Tumors contain subclones—distinct populations of cells with unique genetic alterations. These subclones may respond differently to therapy, making treatment more challenging. For instance, a single tumor might harbor subclones resistant to chemotherapy while others remain sensitive, leading to treatment failure and relapse.

Epigenetic Variability

Beyond genetic changes, tumors exhibit epigenetic heterogeneity. Epigenetic modifications, such as DNA methylation and histone modifications, influence gene expression without altering the DNA sequence. These changes are dynamic and can be driven by environmental factors, further contributing to tumor complexity.

Microenvironmental Influence

Tumor cells interact with their microenvironment, including immune cells, stromal cells, blood vessels, and extracellular matrix. These interactions create additional layers of heterogeneity, influencing tumor growth, metastasis, and resistance to therapy.

Temporal Dynamics

Tumor heterogeneity is not static. As cancer progresses, the composition and behavior of subclones change, often under selective pressures such as immune surveillance or therapy. This dynamic nature makes tracking and targeting tumors more challenging.

Clonal Evolution: The Driver of Cancer Progression

Clonal evolution is the process by which cancer cells accumulate genetic and epigenetic changes over time, leading to the emergence of new subclonal populations. This concept, rooted in Darwinian principles, involves competition, selection, and adaptation within the tumor ecosystem.

Initiation

Clonal evolution begins with a single cell acquiring a driver mutation, which confers a growth or survival advantage. This mutated cell proliferates, giving rise to a dominant clone.

Expansion

As the dominant clone grows, it accumulates additional mutations. Some of these changes provide further advantages, while others are neutral or even deleterious. During this phase, subclonal diversity increases.

Selective Pressures

The tumor microenvironment and external factors, such as treatment, act as selective pressures. Subclones that can adapt to these pressures survive and expand, while others diminish.

For example, therapy-resistant subclones may emerge under chemotherapy, leading to relapse.

Metastasis

In advanced stages, some subclones acquire mutations enabling them to invade surrounding tissues and spread to distant organs. These metastatic subclones often have distinct characteristics from the primary tumor, complicating treatment strategies.

Multi-Omics: Unraveling Complexity

The multi-omics revolution provides powerful tools to study tumor heterogeneity and clonal evolution comprehensively. By integrating data from multiple biological layers, scientists can gain a more detailed understanding of tumor biology.

Genomics

Whole-genome and whole-exome sequencing reveal the mutational landscape of tumors, identifying driver mutations and subclonal populations.

Techniques like single-cell sequencing allow for high-resolution analysis of intra-tumor heterogeneity.

Transcriptomics

RNA sequencing uncovers gene expression profiles, highlighting active pathways in different subclones. This information is crucial for identifying therapeutic targets and understanding tumor behavior.

Epigenomics

Mapping epigenetic modifications sheds light on regulatory changes driving clonal evolution. For instance, altered DNA methylation patterns can silence tumor suppressor genes or activate oncogenes.

Proteomics and Metabolomics

Proteomics studies the functional output of genes, while metabolomics examines metabolic alterations in tumors. Together, they provide insights into the biochemical processes fueling tumor growth and survival.

Spatial and Temporal Dynamics

Advanced imaging and spatial transcriptomics enable researchers to study how tumor heterogeneity evolves over time and space. This approach reveals how subclones interact with their microenvironment and respond to therapy.

Implications for Cancer Treatment

Understanding tumor heterogeneity and clonal evolution has profound implications for cancer therapy. Traditional treatments often target the dominant clone, leaving resistant subclones to repopulate the tumor.

Multi-omics approaches help identify these resistant subclones early, enabling personalized therapies tailored to the tumor's unique composition.

The Multi-Omics Revolution

Combination Therapies

By targeting multiple subclones simultaneously, combination therapies can minimize the risk of resistance. Multi-omics data guide the selection of synergistic drug combinations.

Adaptive Strategies

Real-time monitoring of clonal evolution allows for adaptive treatment strategies. For instance, therapy can be adjusted to target emerging resistant subclones.

Immunotherapy

Multi-omics analyses help identify neoantigens—unique markers on tumor cells enhancing the efficacy of immunotherapies like checkpoint inhibitors and CAR-T cells.

Future Directions

The integration of multi-omics data with artificial intelligence and machine learning is poised to revolutionize cancer research further.

Predictive models based on clonal evolution patterns may enable early detection of resistance and more effective intervention strategies.

Moreover, as technologies become more accessible, the benefits of precision oncology could extend to broader patient populations.

In conclusion, tumor heterogeneity and clonal evolution exemplify the complexity of cancer biology.

The multi-omics revolution offers unprecedented opportunities to decode this complexity, paving the way for more precise, effective, and personalized cancer therapies.

Drug Resistance Mechanisms

Drug resistance is one of the most formidable challenges in cancer research and treatment. Despite significant advancements in oncology, the phenomenon of drug resistance often renders therapies less effective or completely ineffective, leading to treatment failure and disease progression. Understanding the mechanisms behind drug resistance is critical for designing more effective treatment strategies and improving patient outcomes.

Cancer cells are remarkably adaptable, utilizing a variety of mechanisms to evade the effects of therapeutic agents. These mechanisms can broadly be categorized into intrinsic and acquired resistance. Intrinsic resistance refers to pre-existing characteristics of cancer cells that make them less susceptible to treatment. In contrast, acquired resistance develops over time as cancer cells adapt to the selective pressures imposed by therapy.

1. Genetic Alterations and Mutations

One primary mechanism of drug resistance involves genetic mutations in cancer cells. These mutations can alter the drug's target, rendering it less effective. For example, in lung cancer, mutations in the epidermal growth factor receptor (EGFR) can lead to resistance against EGFR-targeted therapies. Similarly, mutations in the BCR-ABL gene in chronic myeloid leukemia (CML) can result in resistance to tyrosine kinase inhibitors like imatinib.

Cancer cells may also activate alternative signaling pathways to bypass the inhibited target. For instance, if one pathway critical for cancer cell survival is blocked by a drug, cells may upregulate a different pathway to continue proliferating. This redundancy in signaling pathways highlights the complexity of cancer biology and the need for combination therapies that target multiple pathways simultaneously.

2. Drug Efflux and Reduced Uptake

Another significant mechanism of drug resistance is the ability of cancer cells to reduce the intracellular concentration of drugs. This is often achieved by upregulating efflux pumps, such as P-glycoprotein (P-gp), which actively transport drugs out of the cell. Overexpression of efflux pumps decreases drug accumulation within cancer cells, lowering their effectiveness.

In some cases, cancer cells may also reduce the expression of transporters responsible for drug uptake. Without sufficient uptake, even highly potent drugs cannot reach their therapeutic targets within the cells.

3. Drug Metabolism and Detoxification

Cancer cells can alter drug metabolism to neutralize the therapeutic agent. Enzymes such as cytochrome P450 play a significant role in this process. Increased activity of these enzymes can convert active drugs into inactive metabolites, reducing their efficacy.

Additionally, cancer cells can enhance their antioxidant defenses to counteract oxidative stress induced by certain drugs. For example, drugs like cisplatin generate reactive oxygen species (ROS) to damage cancer cells. However, increased production of antioxidants like glutathione can neutralize ROS, enabling cancer cells to survive treatment.

4. Tumor Microenvironment

The tumor microenvironment (TME) is a dynamic network of cancer cells, stromal cells, immune cells, and extracellular matrix components. The TME can significantly influence drug response and resistance.

Hypoxic conditions within the TME, for example, can promote the expression of genes associated with drug resistance.

Cancer-associated fibroblasts (CAFs) and immune cells can also secrete growth factors and cytokines that shield cancer cells from therapeutic agents.

Furthermore, the dense extracellular matrix in some tumors can act as a physical barrier, preventing drugs from effectively penetrating the tumor.

5. Epigenetic Modifications

Epigenetic changes, such as DNA methylation, histone modification, and non-coding RNA regulation, play a pivotal role in drug resistance.

These changes can alter gene expression without affecting the DNA sequence, allowing cancer cells to adapt to therapy.

For example, hypermethylation of tumor suppressor genes can silence their expression, enabling cancer cells to survive and proliferate despite treatment.

Epigenetic plasticity also allows cancer cells to switch between different cellular states, such as from an epithelial to a mesenchymal state (epithelial-mesenchymal transition, or EMT).

This transition is associated with increased invasiveness, metastasis, and resistance to therapy.

6. Immune Evasion

Immune checkpoint inhibitors, such as anti-PD-1/PD-L1 therapies, have revolutionized cancer treatment. However, some tumors develop resistance by creating an immunosuppressive environment. Cancer cells can upregulate immune checkpoint molecules or recruit regulatory T cells (Tregs) and myeloid-derived suppressor cells (MDSCs) to suppress the anti-tumor immune response.

7. Cancer Stem Cells

Cancer stem cells (CSCs) are a subpopulation of tumor cells with the ability to self-renew and differentiate. These cells are often inherently resistant to conventional therapies due to their quiescent nature, high expression of efflux pumps, and enhanced DNA repair mechanisms. CSCs are thought to play a critical role in tumor relapse and metastasis.

8. Strategies to Overcome Drug Resistance

Addressing drug resistance requires a multifaceted approach.

Strategies include:

Combination Therapies: Targeting multiple pathways simultaneously to prevent compensatory mechanisms.

Precision Medicine: Using genetic and molecular profiling to tailor treatments to individual patients.

Epigenetic Therapy: Reversing resistance through drugs that modify epigenetic changes.

Overcoming the TME: Developing therapies that target stromal components or improve drug delivery.

The integration of advanced technologies, such as multi-omics approaches (genomics, transcriptomics, proteomics, and metabolomics), is providing unprecedented insights into the complex mechanisms of drug resistance. By understanding these processes at a systems level, researchers can develop innovative strategies to counteract resistance and improve the efficacy of cancer therapies.

The fight against drug resistance in cancer is far from over, but with continued research and technological advancements, there is hope for more effective and durable treatments.

11. Neuroscience

Cellular Diversity in the Brain

The human brain is an intricate and complex organ, composed of an astonishing array of cell types. This cellular diversity is fundamental to the brain's ability to process information, regulate body functions, and generate behaviors. Understanding this diversity has been significantly advanced by the multi-omics revolution, which integrates different layers of biological information to provide a comprehensive view of cellular identity, function, and interaction.

The Foundation of Cellular Diversity

The brain's cellular composition is traditionally divided into two main categories: neurons and glial cells. Neurons are specialized for communication through electrical and chemical signals, forming the basis of neural networks that drive cognition, emotion, and motor control. Glial cells, once thought to be mere support cells, are now recognized as active participants in brain function. These include astrocytes, microglia, and oligodendrocytes, each with distinct roles in maintaining the brain's homeostasis, immune defense, and neural connectivity.

However, this binary classification only scratches the surface. Within these broad categories lies a spectrum of subtypes, each with unique gene expression patterns, morphologies, and physiological roles. For instance, excitatory and inhibitory neurons differ in their neurotransmitter profiles, connectivity, and contributions to neural circuits.

Similarly, astrocytes in different brain regions exhibit specialized functions tailored to local neural environments.

The Multi-Omics Revolution

The Multi-Omics Approach to Cellular Diversity

The advent of multi-omics technologies has transformed our ability to explore cellular diversity. These approaches include genomics, transcriptomics, proteomics, epigenomics, and metabolomics, each offering insights into different aspects of cellular identity and function.

Single-cell Transcriptomics: This technique allows researchers to analyze gene expression at the level of individual cells. By applying single-cell RNA sequencing (scRNA-seq), scientists have uncovered dozens of neuron and glial subtypes, each with distinct expression profiles.

These studies reveal how gene activity varies across cells, providing a molecular basis for functional specialization.

Epigenomics: Epigenetic modifications, such as DNA methylation and histone modifications, influence how genes are expressed without altering the underlying DNA sequence.

Epigenomic studies have shown how cellular identity is shaped during development and maintained throughout life, offering clues to how environmental factors and aging affect brain cells.

Spatial Transcriptomics: This technology maps gene expression to specific locations within the brain.

By combining spatial data with single-cell analyses, researchers can correlate cellular diversity with the anatomical and functional architecture of the brain.

Proteomics and Metabolomics: These approaches study the proteins and metabolites that define cellular function. While gene expression provides a blueprint, proteomics and metabolomics reveal the functional outcomes, shedding light on how diverse brain cells respond to stimuli and interact with each other.

Implications of Cellular Diversity

The brain's cellular diversity is not a static feature; it changes across the lifespan and in response to various conditions. For example, during development, neural progenitor cells differentiate into diverse neuronal and glial subtypes.

This process is tightly regulated by genetic and epigenetic mechanisms, ensuring proper brain formation and function.

In adulthood, cellular diversity underpins the brain's plasticity—the ability to adapt to experiences and recover from injury. Astrocytes and microglia, for instance, play critical roles in synaptic remodeling and immune responses.

The dynamic interplay among cell types is essential for maintaining cognitive function and overall brain health.

In disease states, this diversity can become a double-edged sword. Many neurological and psychiatric disorders are linked to disruptions in specific cell populations. For instance, the loss of dopaminergic neurons in Parkinson's disease or the hyperactivation of microglia in neurodegenerative diseases highlights the importance of understanding cellular diversity. Multi-omics studies have begun to identify molecular signatures associated with these conditions, paving the way for targeted therapies.

The Road Ahead

Despite remarkable progress, much remains to be discovered about the brain's cellular landscape. Future research aims to integrate multi-omics data with advanced imaging, computational modeling, and functional assays to construct a holistic understanding of brain function. These efforts could revolutionize neuroscience, offering insights into the mechanisms of learning, memory, and behavior while also providing new avenues for treating brain disorders.

The Multi-Omics Revolution

The multi-omics revolution underscores the complexity of the brain's cellular diversity and its importance for health and disease.

By unraveling the molecular and functional characteristics of diverse brain cell types, we gain not only a deeper understanding of this extraordinary organ but also the tools to address its vulnerabilities.

In this pursuit, the integration of cutting-edge technologies promises to unlock the secrets of the brain, advancing both science and medicine.

Pathways in Neurodegenerative Diseases

Neurodegenerative diseases, such as Alzheimer's disease (AD), Parkinson's disease (PD), Huntington's disease (HD), and amyotrophic lateral sclerosis (ALS), represent a significant challenge in medicine due to their complex and multifactorial nature.

These conditions are characterized by the progressive loss of structure and function of neurons, leading to cognitive and motor impairments.

Recent advances in multi-omics technologies—encompassing genomics, transcriptomics, proteomics, metabolomics, and epigenomics—have provided unprecedented insights into the molecular pathways underlying these diseases.

By integrating data from multiple omics layers, researchers are uncovering the intricate networks and pathways that drive disease progression, opening avenues for early diagnosis, targeted therapies, and precision medicine.

Key Molecular Pathways in Neurodegenerative Diseases

Amyloid and Tau Pathways in Alzheimer's Disease

In Alzheimer's disease, two hallmark protein abnormalities dominate: amyloid-beta plaques and tau tangles. Genomic studies have identified mutations in the APP, PSEN1, and PSEN2 genes that influence amyloid precursor protein processing, leading to amyloid-beta accumulation.

Transcriptomic and proteomic analyses further reveal dysregulation in tau phosphorylation pathways, which destabilize microtubules and impair neuronal transport.

Multi-omics approaches highlight the interplay between amyloid and tau pathways, suggesting feedback loops and shared regulators that exacerbate neuronal toxicity.

Alpha-Synuclein and Dopaminergic Pathways in Parkinson's Disease

Parkinson's disease is characterized by the aggregation of alpha-synuclein into Lewy bodies and the selective loss of dopaminergic neurons in the substantia nigra.

Genomic studies link mutations in genes such as SNCA (encoding alpha-synuclein), LRRK2, and PARKIN to familial forms of PD.

Proteomic profiling has identified alpha-synuclein interactomes and post-translational modifications that drive its aggregation.

Metabolomic analyses reveal alterations in dopamine biosynthesis and mitochondrial pathways, emphasizing the role of cellular energy dysregulation in PD pathogenesis.

Huntingtin Pathways in Huntington's Disease

Huntington's disease results from an expanded CAG repeat in the HTT gene, leading to a toxic gain-of-function in the huntingtin protein. Transcriptomic studies have shown widespread gene expression changes due to the interaction of mutant huntingtin with transcriptional regulators. Proteomics has uncovered dysregulated protein-protein interactions, while metabolomics highlights disrupted energy metabolism, especially in the striatum.

Multi-omics integration sheds light on the connections between mutant huntingtin, oxidative stress, and neuroinflammation, offering potential targets for therapeutic intervention.

TDP-43 and SOD1 Pathways in Amyotrophic Lateral Sclerosis

ALS involves the aggregation of misfolded proteins such as TDP-43 and mutations in genes like SOD1, C9orf72, and FUS. Genomic and epigenomic analyses reveal diverse genetic contributions, including repeat expansions, point mutations, and regulatory changes. Proteomics has illuminated the role of TDP-43 in RNA metabolism and stress granule dynamics.

Metabolomic studies highlight disruptions in energy homeostasis and lipid metabolism. Multi-omics approaches reveal that ALS pathology involves a convergence of genetic, proteostatic, and metabolic stress pathways.

Common Pathways Across Neurodegenerative Diseases

Despite their distinct clinical features, neurodegenerative diseases share common molecular pathways, including:

Oxidative Stress: Reactive oxygen species (ROS) accumulation damages proteins, lipids, and DNA, contributing to neuronal death.

Multi-omics studies link oxidative stress to mitochondrial dysfunction, impaired proteostasis, and neuroinflammation.

Neuroinflammation: Chronic activation of microglia and astrocytes leads to the release of pro-inflammatory cytokines, exacerbating neuronal damage.

Transcriptomics and metabolomics highlight key mediators and metabolic shifts in inflammatory pathways.

Autophagy and Proteostasis: Impaired clearance of misfolded proteins is a unifying feature.

Proteomic analyses have revealed disruptions in the autophagy-lysosome pathway across multiple neurodegenerative diseases.

Synaptic Dysfunction: Loss of synaptic integrity is an early event. Multi-omics studies uncover alterations in synaptic proteins, lipid composition, and signaling pathways that precede neuronal loss.

Implications for Therapeutics

Multi-omics technologies are transforming our understanding of neurodegenerative diseases by identifying novel biomarkers, therapeutic targets, and molecular subtypes of diseases.

For instance:

Biomarker Discovery: Integrating proteomic and metabolomic data has led to the identification of cerebrospinal fluid and blood biomarkers for early diagnosis, such as neurofilament light chain in ALS and phosphorylated tau in AD.

Targeted Therapies: Genomic and transcriptomic insights are driving the development of gene therapies, such as antisense oligonucleotides for HD and ALS.

Precision Medicine: Multi-omics approaches enable patient stratification based on molecular profiles, allowing for personalized treatment strategies.

The Multi-Omics Revolution

Future Directions

The field is moving toward integrating single-cell omics and spatial transcriptomics to study neuronal and glial heterogeneity.

Advanced computational tools and machine learning are essential for interpreting the vast datasets generated by multi-omics studies.

Collaboration across disciplines will be crucial for translating these findings into clinical practice.

In conclusion, the multi-omics revolution is unraveling the complexities of neurodegenerative diseases, providing a comprehensive view of their molecular underpinnings.

By mapping the pathways that drive these diseases, researchers are paving the way for breakthroughs in diagnostics, therapeutics, and prevention, bringing hope to millions affected by these devastating conditions.

12. Immunology

Single-cell Profiling of Immune Responses

The immune system is a complex network of cells and molecules designed to protect the body from pathogens and maintain homeostasis. Over the years, scientific advancements have unraveled many aspects of immune function.

Yet, understanding immune responses at the level of individual cells has remained challenging due to the immense diversity and dynamic nature of immune cells.

This is where single-cell profiling has revolutionized immunology, offering unprecedented insights into the behavior, identity, and interaction of immune cells.

What is Single-Cell Profiling?

Single-cell profiling refers to the ability to analyze individual cells' genetic, epigenetic, proteomic, or metabolic properties. Traditional methods, such as bulk sequencing, average signals from millions of cells, obscuring the heterogeneity and unique functions of specific cell subpopulations.

In contrast, single-cell techniques capture the individuality of each cell, revealing their distinct states and roles within a larger system.

This approach has become especially valuable in studying the immune system, which consists of diverse cell types like T cells, B cells, macrophages, and dendritic cells. Each of these cell types can exhibit a wide range of behaviors depending on the context, such as during infection, autoimmunity, or cancer.

The Multi-Omics Revolution

Tools and Techniques in Single-Cell Profiling
Several powerful technologies enable single-cell profiling, including:

Single-Cell RNA Sequencing (scRNA-seq): This technique analyzes gene expression patterns in individual cells, providing insights into their functional states and interactions.

For immune cells, scRNA-seq can identify activated T cells, antibody-producing B cells, or inflammatory macrophages during immune responses.

Mass Cytometry (CyTOF): By tagging proteins on cell surfaces with heavy metal isotopes, CyTOF measures the expression of dozens of markers simultaneously.

This technique is particularly useful for characterizing immune cell phenotypes and tracking their changes in response to stimuli.

Single-Cell ATAC Sequencing (scATAC-seq): This method maps open chromatin regions in single cells, revealing regulatory elements that control gene expression. In immune cells, scATAC-seq can uncover how transcription factors shape cell differentiation and activation.

Spatial Transcriptomics: By integrating spatial information, this approach reveals the physical context of immune cells within tissues.

It helps in understanding how immune cells coordinate their responses in specific microenvironments, such as lymph nodes or tumors.

Proteomics and Metabolomics at Single-Cell Resolution: These methods analyze the proteins and metabolites within individual immune cells, shedding light on their functional states and metabolic dependencies.

Applications in Immune Research

Single-cell profiling has dramatically transformed our understanding of immune responses.

Here are some of the key areas where it has made significant contributions:

Deciphering Immune Cell Diversity: The immune system's complexity lies in its diversity. Single-cell profiling has identified previously unknown subsets of immune cells, such as novel T cell populations or macrophage states, and has helped map their roles in health and disease.

Tracking Immune Responses Over Time: Immune responses are dynamic, evolving from activation to resolution. Single-cell techniques allow researchers to monitor how individual cells change during this process. For instance, tracking T cells during viral infections can reveal the emergence of memory cells that provide long-term protection.

Understanding Autoimmune Disorders: In autoimmune diseases, the immune system mistakenly attacks the body's own tissues. Single-cell profiling helps pinpoint which cells are involved, how they become dysregulated, and how therapies can restore balance.

Cancer Immunology: The tumor microenvironment is a battleground between cancer cells and immune cells. Single-cell profiling has been instrumental in identifying exhausted T cells that fail to attack tumors and finding ways to rejuvenate them through immunotherapy.

Infectious Diseases: Single-cell studies have revealed how different immune cells respond to pathogens like viruses, bacteria, or parasites. For example, during COVID-19, scRNA-seq was used to study immune responses to SARS-CoV-2, providing insights into disease severity and treatment targets.

The Multi-Omics Revolution

Vaccine Development: Understanding how vaccines stimulate immune cells at a single-cell level has improved vaccine design. Researchers can identify the specific B and T cells activated by a vaccine, ensuring robust and long-lasting protection.

Challenges and Future Directions

While single-cell profiling offers remarkable insights, it also comes with challenges. The techniques can be technically demanding, requiring sophisticated equipment and bioinformatics expertise.

Additionally, the vast amount of data generated needs careful interpretation to avoid overgeneralizations or misinterpretations.

Looking forward, advances in multi-omics approaches will integrate data from genomics, transcriptomics, proteomics, and metabolomics at the single-cell level. This holistic view will provide a deeper understanding of immune regulation. Moreover, improvements in spatial resolution will allow researchers to study how immune cells interact with other cell types in their native environments.

Single-cell profiling has opened a new era in immunology, transforming our understanding of immune responses at an unprecedented resolution. By revealing the unique characteristics and behaviors of individual cells, it has provided critical insights into health and disease.

As technologies continue to evolve, single-cell profiling will undoubtedly drive the next wave of discoveries, paving the way for personalized immunotherapies, better vaccines, and innovative treatments for immune-related disorders.

This multi-omics revolution is not just a leap in technology but a transformative lens through which we understand life at its most intricate level.

Implications for Vaccine Development

The field of vaccine development has witnessed transformative advancements in recent decades, but the advent of multi-omics has taken this evolution to unprecedented heights.

Multi-omics—an integrative approach combining genomics, transcriptomics, proteomics, metabolomics, and epigenomics—offers an unparalleled depth of understanding about the complex biological systems at play in immunity.

This revolution not only accelerates vaccine discovery but also optimizes their design, effectiveness, and accessibility.

Understanding the Host-Pathogen Interaction

At the heart of vaccine development lies a fundamental question: how does the human body respond to pathogens? Multi-omics provides a comprehensive map of host-pathogen interactions.

For instance, genomics identifies specific genetic predispositions to infections, helping scientists pinpoint target populations for vaccination.

Transcriptomics, which studies RNA expression, reveals how immune-related genes are activated in response to pathogens, offering clues to effective immune defense mechanisms.

By integrating proteomics—the study of proteins—researchers can examine the antigens that pathogens use to invade host cells. This allows for the identification of highly specific targets for vaccine design. Metabolomics and lipidomics further elucidate how metabolic pathways and lipid interactions influence immunity.

Together, these layers of data provide a panoramic view of how the body recognizes and fights infectious agents.

The Multi-Omics Revolution

Accelerating Antigen Discovery

Traditional vaccine development relies heavily on cultivating pathogens in laboratory settings and isolating antigens through trial and error. Multi-omics has drastically reduced the time required for this phase. Genomic sequencing of pathogens allows researchers to identify antigen candidates directly from the pathogen's DNA.

For example, reverse vaccinology, a technique powered by genomics, was instrumental in developing the meningococcal B vaccine by predicting antigenic proteins from the bacterium's genome.

Proteomics enhances this process by characterizing the three-dimensional structures of proteins, helping to identify epitopes—the specific parts of an antigen that are recognized by the immune system. This streamlined antigen discovery process not only improves efficiency but also ensures a higher probability of vaccine efficacy.

Personalizing Vaccination Strategies

A significant leap offered by multi-omics is the potential for personalized vaccines. Variations in genetic and epigenetic factors mean that immune responses to vaccines differ among individuals. Multi-omics enables the identification of biomarkers that predict vaccine responsiveness, allowing for the customization of vaccine formulations or dosing strategies to maximize effectiveness.

For instance, studies have shown that age-related changes in epigenetic markers and metabolic profiles can influence immune responses.

By integrating epigenomics and metabolomics data, researchers can tailor vaccines for specific populations, such as infants, the elderly, or immunocompromised individuals.

Tackling Emerging and Re-Emerging Infectious Diseases

Emerging infectious diseases like COVID-19 underscore the importance of rapid vaccine development. Multi-omics platforms are indispensable tools in the fight against such outbreaks.

enables real-time tracking of pathogen evolution, identifying new variants that may evade existing vaccines.

The integration of transcriptomics and proteomics helps elucidate the mechanisms of immune evasion and guide the design of next-generation vaccines.

Furthermore, multi-omics contributes to vaccine development for re-emerging diseases, such as tuberculosis, where traditional vaccines have shown limited efficacy.

By uncovering complex immune pathways and identifying new antigenic targets, multi-omics offers hope for more effective solutions.

Enhancing Vaccine Safety and Efficacy

One of the challenges in vaccine development is ensuring both safety and efficacy. Multi-omics plays a critical role in de-risking this process. For example, proteomics and metabolomics can identify off-target effects of vaccine candidates by revealing unintended interactions with the host's biological systems. This enables the design of safer vaccines with minimal side effects.

Simultaneously, transcriptomics can monitor immune activation post-vaccination to ensure robust and long-lasting immunity.

By analyzing immune signatures in vaccinated individuals, researchers can refine vaccine formulations to achieve optimal protection.

The Multi-Omics Revolution

Advancing Adjuvant Development

Adjuvants are substances added to vaccines to enhance immune responses. The selection and design of effective adjuvants have traditionally been a trial-and-error process. Multi-omics revolutionizes this by identifying molecular pathways activated by existing adjuvants, paving the way for the design of more targeted and potent alternatives.

For instance, transcriptomics and metabolomics can reveal how specific adjuvants influence cytokine production and metabolic reprogramming of immune cells.

These insights guide the development of novel adjuvants that synergize with vaccine antigens for maximum efficacy.

The Role of Artificial Intelligence and Big Data

The vast amounts of data generated by multi-omics require advanced computational tools for analysis. Artificial intelligence (AI) and machine learning algorithms are integral to identifying patterns and predicting outcomes from multi-omics datasets.

In vaccine development, AI-driven multi-omics platforms can predict antigenicity, immune response profiles, and potential adverse effects, accelerating the pathway from discovery to deployment.

Bridging the Gap in Global Vaccine Equity

Multi-omics also holds promise for addressing global disparities in vaccine access. By streamlining antigen discovery and manufacturing processes, multi-omics reduces costs, making vaccines more affordable.

Additionally, the integration of multi-omics data from diverse populations ensures that vaccines are effective across different genetic backgrounds and environmental conditions.

The multi-omics revolution is not just a technological advancement; it represents a paradigm shift in vaccine development.

By unraveling the intricacies of host-pathogen interactions, streamlining antigen discovery, enabling personalized strategies, and enhancing safety and efficacy, multi-omics offers a comprehensive toolkit for tackling infectious diseases.

As this field continues to evolve, its integration with artificial intelligence and big data analytics promises to usher in a new era of precision vaccines, saving lives and improving global health outcomes.

13. Regenerative Medicine

Single-Cell Insights into Stem Cell Biology

Stem cell biology has become a cornerstone of regenerative medicine, offering the promise of repairing damaged tissues and organs by harnessing the body's intrinsic ability to regenerate.

The advent of single-cell multi-omics has transformed our understanding of stem cells, shedding light on their complex biology at an unprecedented level.

This breakthrough allows researchers to analyze the molecular makeup of individual cells, revealing intricate details that were previously obscured by bulk cell analysis.

The Role of Stem Cells in Regenerative Medicine

Stem cells are unique because of their ability to differentiate into specialized cell types and their capacity for self-renewal.

These properties make them invaluable in regenerative medicine, where they are used to treat conditions ranging from neurodegenerative disorders to cardiac disease and diabetes.

However, the effectiveness of stem cell-based therapies hinges on a deep understanding of their biology.

Factors such as how stem cells maintain their pluripotency (the ability to develop into multiple cell types), how they decide to differentiate, and how their microenvironment influences these decisions are critical to the success of such therapies.

Why Single-Cell Analysis Matters

Traditional methods of studying stem cells often involved bulk analysis, where populations of cells are studied together. While this approach provided valuable insights, it obscured the heterogeneity inherent in stem cell populations. Not all stem cells within a given sample behave identically; they may exist in different states of activation, differentiation potential, or gene expression. Bulk analysis averages these differences, leading to incomplete or misleading conclusions.

Single-cell analysis addresses this limitation by examining individual cells, allowing researchers to dissect the variability within stem cell populations. This has proven essential for identifying rare subpopulations of cells with unique regenerative capabilities and understanding how cellular diversity contributes to tissue regeneration and repair.

Single-Cell Multi-Omics: A Game-Changer

Single-cell multi-omics combines multiple layers of biological data, such as genomics, transcriptomics, epigenomics, and proteomics, from individual cells.

This approach offers a comprehensive view of stem cell biology by integrating information about:

Gene Expression (Transcriptomics): By analyzing RNA molecules in single cells, scientists can determine which genes are active at any given time. This is crucial for understanding how stem cells transition from a pluripotent state to specialized cell types.

Epigenetic Regulation (Epigenomics): Epigenetic modifications, such as DNA methylation and histone modifications, play a key role in controlling gene expression. Single-cell epigenomics reveals how these modifications influence stem cell fate.

Protein Activity (Proteomics): Proteins are the functional molecules in cells, driving processes such as signaling and metabolism. Single-cell proteomics helps identify key proteins involved in stem cell differentiation and self-renewal.

Metabolic States (Metabolomics): Metabolic pathways often dictate cellular behavior. Single-cell metabolomics allows researchers to track how energy production and consumption impact stem cell function.

Insights from Single-Cell Studies

Single-cell techniques have already yielded groundbreaking insights into stem cell biology.

For example:

Identifying Stem Cell Niches: Stem cells do not operate in isolation; they are influenced by their microenvironment, or "niche." Single-cell analysis has helped identify the cellular and molecular components of these niches, providing clues on how to recreate optimal conditions for stem cell therapy.

Understanding Stem Cell Plasticity: Stem cells exhibit remarkable plasticity, adapting to different cues to generate diverse cell types. Single-cell studies have uncovered the molecular mechanisms underlying this plasticity, paving the way for more precise control over stem cell differentiation.

Tracking Lineage Commitment: Single-cell lineage tracing techniques have been used to map the differentiation trajectories of stem cells. This has helped in understanding how specific signals guide stem cells to become neurons, muscle cells, or other specialized types.

Detecting Rare Cell States: Rare subpopulations of stem cells with unique regenerative potential have been identified through single-cell analysis. These cells are often critical for effective tissue repair but are overlooked in bulk studies.

Applications in Regenerative Medicine

The insights gained from single-cell studies are being translated into clinical applications.

Some notable examples include:

Improved Cell Therapies: By identifying the most potent stem cells, researchers can enhance the effectiveness of cell-based therapies for conditions such as spinal cord injuries and heart disease.

Drug Screening: Single-cell platforms are used to test how potential drugs affect stem cells, accelerating the development of regenerative treatments.

Personalized Medicine: Single-cell analysis enables the development of personalized regenerative therapies tailored to the unique cellular landscape of individual patients.

Organoid Development: Organoids—miniature, lab-grown versions of organs—are being used to study disease and test treatments. Single-cell techniques ensure that these organoids closely mimic the cellular complexity of real tissues.

Challenges and Future Directions

Despite its promise, single-cell multi-omics is not without challenges.

The techniques are technically demanding, require sophisticated computational tools, and generate massive amounts of data that must be carefully interpreted.

Moreover, translating insights from single-cell studies into clinical therapies requires rigorous validation and regulatory approval.

The Multi-Omics Revolution

Future advancements in technology are likely to address these challenges, making single-cell multi-omics more accessible and scalable.

Emerging methods such as spatial transcriptomics, which combines single-cell analysis with spatial information, promise to provide even deeper insights into how stem cells interact within their native environments.

Single-cell multi-omics has revolutionized stem cell research, offering unprecedented insights into the molecular mechanisms that drive regeneration.

By unraveling the complexities of individual cells, this approach is paving the way for transformative advances in regenerative medicine.

As the technology continues to evolve, it holds the potential to unlock new therapeutic possibilities, bringing us closer to the goal of repairing and regenerating tissues with precision and efficiency.

Tissue Engineering Applications

Tissue engineering, a cornerstone of regenerative medicine, represents a groundbreaking approach to repairing, replacing, or regenerating damaged tissues and organs. This interdisciplinary field integrates principles from biology, engineering, and materials science to create functional tissues capable of restoring normal function in diseased or injured parts of the body.

The advent of multi-omics technologies—genomics, transcriptomics, proteomics, and metabolomics—has further propelled this field, enabling researchers to unravel complex biological processes and design more effective tissue engineering strategies.

The Foundations of Tissue Engineering

At its core, tissue engineering involves three primary components: scaffolds, cells, and bioactive signals. Scaffolds are three-dimensional structures that provide a physical framework for cells to adhere, proliferate, and differentiate.

Cells, often sourced from the patient (autologous), donors (allogeneic), or stem cell lines, are seeded onto these scaffolds. Bioactive signals, such as growth factors or cytokines, guide cell behavior and tissue formation.

Together, these elements mimic the natural environment of tissues, encouraging regeneration in a controlled and predictable manner.

Advancements Through Multi-Omics

Multi-omics technologies have revolutionized our understanding of tissue dynamics and the microenvironment.

Genomics reveals the genetic blueprint of tissues, helping identify mutations or genetic predispositions affecting regeneration.

Transcriptomics captures the gene expression profiles during tissue repair, offering insights into the molecular pathways active in different stages of regeneration.

Proteomics sheds light on the proteins involved in cell signaling, adhesion, and extracellular matrix formation, while metabolomics maps the biochemical processes that sustain cellular activity and energy production.

This integrated knowledge helps researchers tailor tissue engineering approaches to individual patients, fostering the emergence of personalized regenerative therapies.

The Multi-Omics Revolution

Applications in Regenerative Medicine

Skin Regeneration

Skin tissue engineering has made remarkable strides in treating burns, chronic wounds, and skin disorders. Bioengineered skin substitutes, such as artificial dermal layers combined with epidermal cells, provide effective solutions for extensive injuries. Multi-omics studies have facilitated the identification of key proteins and growth factors critical for wound healing, leading to more effective scaffold designs and therapeutic strategies.

Bone and Cartilage Repair

Orthopedic applications are among the most prominent areas of tissue engineering. Scaffold materials, such as bioceramics and biodegradable polymers, are employed to support bone and cartilage repair. By analyzing the proteomic and transcriptomic profiles of bone cells, researchers have optimized the use of growth factors like bone morphogenetic proteins (BMPs) to enhance bone regeneration.

Similarly, for cartilage repair, chondrocytes and mesenchymal stem cells (MSCs) are used in combination with hydrogels to regenerate cartilage in conditions like osteoarthritis.

Cardiac Tissue Regeneration

Cardiovascular diseases often lead to irreversible damage to the heart muscle. Tissue engineering offers a solution through the creation of cardiac patches composed of biomaterials and cardiomyocytes derived from stem cells. Multi-omics analyses have identified key genes and proteins involved in cardiomyocyte differentiation and maturation, enabling the development of functional cardiac tissues.

These advancements hold promise for patients recovering from myocardial infarction or other cardiac disorders.

Liver Tissue Engineering

Liver failure poses significant challenges due to the organ's complex structure and functions. Advances in tissue engineering aim to recreate functional liver tissues using hepatocytes or liver organoids. Metabolomics has been instrumental in understanding the metabolic demands of liver cells, guiding the design of bioreactors and scaffolds that mimic the liver's microenvironment. These engineered tissues may eventually serve as an alternative to liver transplantation.

Neural Tissue Regeneration

Regenerating neural tissue is particularly challenging due to the intricacy of the nervous system. Tissue engineering approaches involve the use of biomaterial scaffolds infused with neurotrophic factors to guide axonal growth and synapse formation. Transcriptomic and proteomic studies have provided valuable insights into the molecular cues that promote neural regeneration, aiding in the development of treatments for spinal cord injuries, neurodegenerative diseases, and stroke recovery.

Challenges and Future Directions

Despite its remarkable progress, tissue engineering faces several challenges. One major hurdle is achieving vascularization within engineered tissues to ensure adequate oxygen and nutrient supply. Multi-omics research has highlighted key signaling pathways and molecules involved in angiogenesis, paving the way for innovations in creating pre-vascularized tissues.

Immune rejection is another concern, especially when using allogeneic cells. Genomic and proteomic tools are helping scientists develop immune-evasive or immune-compatible biomaterials and cells.

Moreover, integrating artificial intelligence (AI) with multi-omics data promises to accelerate the design and testing of tissue engineering constructs.

The Multi-Omics Revolution

Looking forward, the field is shifting towards the development of fully functional organs.

Bioprinting technologies, combined with omics-driven insights, are enabling the precise layering of cells and biomaterials to recreate the architecture of organs like kidneys, lungs, and the heart.

This could eventually address the global shortage of organ donors.

Tissue engineering, bolstered by multi-omics technologies, is transforming regenerative medicine by offering innovative solutions to some of the most pressing healthcare challenges.

By bridging the gap between biological understanding and engineering ingenuity, this field holds the potential to restore hope and health to millions worldwide.

As researchers continue to refine these techniques and overcome existing barriers, the dream of regenerating complex tissues and organs moves closer to becoming a reality.

14. Microbiome Studies

Single-Cell Analysis of Host-Microbe Interactions

The human body is a bustling ecosystem, home to trillions of microorganisms that play critical roles in health and disease. From the gut to the skin, microbes interact with human cells, shaping physiological processes in ways that are both profound and intricate.

While the relationship between hosts and microbes has long been studied, traditional approaches often failed to capture the granularity of these interactions.

Single-cell analysis has emerged as a revolutionary tool, offering unprecedented insights into the molecular dialogues between individual host cells and microbial partners.

The Importance of Host-Microbe Interactions

Host-microbe interactions are fundamental to the survival and function of multicellular organisms. Microbes contribute to digestion, immune regulation, and even mental health, while the host provides a supportive environment for microbial communities.

Disruptions in this balance—known as dysbiosis—can lead to a range of diseases, including inflammatory bowel disease, obesity, and autoimmune disorders.

Studying these interactions at the single-cell level enables researchers to dissect the specific contributions of individual cells and microbes, revealing dynamics that are masked in bulk analyses.

The Multi-Omics Revolution

Single-Cell Analysis: A Game-Changer

Traditional microbiological techniques often rely on averages across populations of cells, which can obscure important variations.

For example, two seemingly identical host cells may respond very differently to the same microbial stimulus. Single-cell analysis circumvents this limitation by examining the transcriptome, proteome, metabolome, or epigenome of individual cells.

This approach uncovers cellular heterogeneity and provides a clearer picture of how specific cells interact with microbes.

Recent advances in single-cell technologies, such as single-cell RNA sequencing (scRNA-seq) and spatial transcriptomics, have made it possible to study host-microbe interactions in unprecedented detail.

These tools allow researchers to:

Identify Cellular Subpopulations: In a tissue like the gut, single-cell analysis can distinguish between different types of epithelial cells, immune cells, and microbial residents, highlighting their unique roles in maintaining homeostasis.

Map Spatial Relationships: Spatial transcriptomics integrates gene expression data with tissue architecture, revealing how host cells are physically arranged relative to microbial communities.

Capture Dynamic Interactions: Single-cell approaches can track how individual cells change over time in response to microbial cues, offering insights into processes like immune activation and tissue repair.

Insights Gained from Single-Cell Analysis

1. Gut Microbiota and Immune Responses

The gut is a primary site of host-microbe interactions, housing a diverse microbial community that influences immune system development.

Single-cell studies have revealed that certain immune cells, such as macrophages and dendritic cells, exhibit distinct transcriptional profiles depending on the microbes they encounter.

For example, single-cell RNA sequencing has shown how specific bacterial species modulate T-cell differentiation, leading to pro-inflammatory or anti-inflammatory states.

2. Microbial Influence on Tissue Repair

In the gut lining, epithelial cells are constantly renewed to maintain a barrier against microbial invasion. Single-cell analysis has uncovered that some bacterial metabolites directly signal to epithelial stem cells, promoting their proliferation and differentiation.

This interaction is critical for tissue repair after injury and provides a new perspective on how the microbiome supports host health.

3. Skin Microbiome and Host Defense

The skin microbiome acts as a protective shield, modulating the activity of immune cells to fend off pathogens. Single-cell studies have identified specific keratinocytes and immune cell subsets that respond uniquely to commensal versus pathogenic microbes.

These findings could inform strategies to enhance skin barrier function in conditions like eczema and psoriasis.

4. Host-Microbe Crosstalk in Diseases

In diseases like inflammatory bowel disease (IBD), single-cell analysis has revealed an imbalance in the interactions between host immune cells and gut microbes. For instance, single-cell profiling has shown that certain bacterial species exacerbate inflammation by interacting with hyperactive immune cells. These insights open the door to targeted therapies that modulate specific host-microbe interactions.

Challenges and Future Directions

Despite its transformative potential, single-cell analysis of host-microbe interactions faces several challenges. For instance, isolating host and microbial cells from complex tissues without disturbing their natural interactions is technically demanding. Additionally, analyzing microbial gene expression at the single-cell level is complicated by the small size and diversity of microbial genomes.

Future developments in multi-omics integration promise to address these challenges. Combining single-cell transcriptomics with proteomics and metabolomics will provide a more comprehensive view of host-microbe interactions. Advances in machine learning will also help decipher the vast datasets generated by single-cell studies, uncovering hidden patterns and predicting functional outcomes.

Implications for Medicine and Biotechnology

Single-cell analysis is not just a tool for academic discovery; it has practical implications for medicine and biotechnology.

For example:

Personalized Medicine: Understanding individual variations in host-microbe interactions could lead to personalized probiotics or dietary interventions tailored to a person's unique microbiome.

Drug Development: Single-cell insights into microbial effects on immune cells can guide the development of microbiome-based therapies for autoimmune diseases.

Synthetic Biology: Researchers can design engineered microbes that interact with host cells in specific ways, offering new solutions for drug delivery and tissue regeneration.

Single-cell analysis is revolutionizing our understanding of host-microbe interactions, uncovering the molecular intricacies of this vital relationship.

By highlighting cellular heterogeneity and dynamic processes, it provides a foundation for novel therapeutic strategies and a deeper appreciation of the complex interplay between human biology and the microbial world.

As the multi-omics revolution progresses, single-cell technologies will undoubtedly remain at the forefront of host-microbe research, driving innovations that transform both science and medicine.

Environmental and Microbiome Studies

The world we inhabit is a complex, interwoven system where every living organism plays a role in maintaining the balance of ecosystems.

Among the most fascinating components of these ecosystems are the microbiomes—communities of microorganisms, such as bacteria, fungi, viruses, and archaea, that coexist with their environments.

Multi-omics approaches, which integrate data from genomics, transcriptomics, proteomics, metabolomics, and more, have revolutionized our understanding of microbiomes and their influence on the environment.

The Multi-Omics Revolution

Decoding Microbiome Complexity with Multi-Omics

Microbiomes thrive in diverse environments, ranging from soil and water to extreme habitats like hot springs and deep-sea hydrothermal vents. These microorganisms are pivotal to ecosystem functions such as nutrient cycling, carbon sequestration, and pollutant degradation. However, studying such complex and dynamic systems has always been a challenge.

With the advent of multi-omics technologies, researchers now have tools to delve deeper into the intricate interactions between microbial communities and their surroundings.

Genomics provides insights into the genetic potential of microbial species, while transcriptomics uncovers active gene expression under specific environmental conditions.

Proteomics and metabolomics offer layers of data on protein activity and metabolite production, shedding light on functional outcomes of microbial processes. Together, these layers create a comprehensive map of how microbiomes interact with and adapt to their environments.

Environmental Applications of Multi-Omics in Microbiome Studies

Soil Health and Agriculture

Soil microbiomes are critical for plant health and agricultural productivity. Multi-omics has enabled researchers to identify key microbial species that promote plant growth, enhance nutrient availability, and suppress pathogens. For example, by analyzing soil samples through metagenomics and metabolomics, scientists can identify microbial pathways responsible for nitrogen fixation—a process vital for sustainable agriculture.

This understanding aids in designing biofertilizers that reduce reliance on chemical inputs, preserving soil quality over the long term.

Water Quality and Aquatic Ecosystems
Aquatic microbiomes influence water quality, biodiversity, and the global carbon cycle. Multi-omics approaches help track microbial responses to pollutants, such as heavy metals or pesticides, and monitor harmful algal blooms.

Metaproteomics and metabolomics reveal how microbial communities metabolize pollutants, offering clues for bioremediation strategies.

Additionally, such studies inform conservation efforts by identifying microbial indicators of ecosystem health in freshwater and marine environments.

Climate Change Mitigation
Microbial communities play a significant role in regulating greenhouse gas emissions. Wetlands, for instance, are hotspots for methane production, while oceans act as major carbon sinks.

Multi-omics techniques allow scientists to understand the metabolic pathways responsible for methane production or carbon sequestration at the microbial level.

By studying these pathways, researchers can explore ways to mitigate greenhouse gas emissions through ecosystem management.

Bioremediation of Pollutants
The capacity of certain microbial species to degrade pollutants such as oil spills, plastics, and toxic chemicals has positioned microbiomes as key players in environmental cleanup.

Multi-omics enables the identification of microbial consortia and their functional capabilities in pollutant degradation.

For instance, transcriptomics can highlight genes activated in response to hydrocarbons, providing a roadmap for optimizing bioremediation efforts.

The Multi-Omics Revolution

The Role of Multi-Omics in Understanding Microbiome Dynamics

Multi-omics approaches also address temporal and spatial dynamics of microbiomes in their environments. Temporal studies track changes in microbial activity over time, revealing how ecosystems respond to seasonal variations, climate change, or anthropogenic disturbances.

Spatial studies map microbial diversity across different habitats, highlighting how local conditions such as pH, temperature, and nutrient availability shape community composition.

For instance, in the Amazon rainforest, multi-omics analyses have uncovered how microbial communities contribute to the decomposition of organic matter and the recycling of nutrients. Similarly, in Arctic permafrost, researchers have identified microbes capable of metabolizing frozen organic carbon, a process with significant implications for understanding global warming feedback loops.

Challenges and Future Directions

Despite its transformative potential, the integration of multi-omics data comes with challenges. High-throughput sequencing and analytical techniques generate vast amounts of data, requiring sophisticated computational tools and bioinformatics expertise. Moreover, connecting multi-omics insights to ecosystem-level processes often requires interdisciplinary collaboration among microbiologists, ecologists, and data scientists.

Future advancements in multi-omics technologies, such as single-cell multi-omics and spatial omics, promise even greater precision in studying microbial interactions. These tools can provide a deeper understanding of how microbiomes respond to stressors, such as pollution or climate change, and help predict the resilience of ecosystems.

Implications for Human and Planetary Health

Microbiomes are not isolated entities; they form the backbone of ecosystems that sustain life on Earth. By unraveling the connections between microbiomes and their environments, multi-omics studies contribute to global sustainability efforts.

They offer solutions for restoring degraded ecosystems, enhancing food security, and combating climate change.

Moreover, understanding environmental microbiomes has implications for human health. Soil and water microbiomes influence the quality of the food we eat and the water we drink.

By ensuring the health of these systems, we indirectly protect our own health and well-being.

In conclusion, the integration of multi-omics into environmental and microbiome studies marks a paradigm shift in how we understand and interact with the natural world.

By decoding the language of microbial life, we gain the knowledge needed to foster harmony between humanity and the ecosystems that support us.

15. Overcoming Technical and Analytical Challenges

Improving Sensitivity and Throughput

The field of multi-omics is rapidly transforming our understanding of biology by integrating data from genomics, transcriptomics, proteomics, metabolomics, and other omics disciplines. This integrative approach holds the promise of unlocking unprecedented insights into complex biological systems, diseases, and personalized medicine. However, achieving this potential requires addressing significant technical and analytical challenges, particularly in improving sensitivity and throughput.

Enhancing Sensitivity in Multi-Omics Studies

Sensitivity in multi-omics refers to the ability to detect low-abundance molecules, whether they are rare proteins, low-expressed genes, or trace metabolites. Many critical biological signals are subtle, requiring advanced methods to identify and quantify these elements accurately.

Here are some approaches to enhance sensitivity:

Advanced Instrumentation: Modern analytical platforms like mass spectrometry (MS) and next-generation sequencing (NGS) have become indispensable tools for multi-omics. Innovations in MS, such as high-resolution and tandem-MS techniques, allow for the detection of minute quantities of proteins and metabolites.

Similarly, ultra-deep sequencing methods in genomics enhance the ability to capture rare genetic variants and low-frequency transcripts.

Optimized Sample Preparation: Effective sensitivity begins at the sample preparation stage. Methods such as microfluidic technologies and laser-capture microdissection enable the isolation of specific cell types or subcellular components, reducing background noise and enhancing the detection of low-abundance molecules.

Amplification Techniques: For low-input samples, amplification methods, like polymerase chain reaction (PCR) for nucleic acids or signal amplification strategies in proteomics, boost the detectability of scarce molecules. These techniques need careful optimization to prevent artifacts and maintain accuracy.

Noise Reduction Strategies: Background noise is a major impediment to sensitivity. Techniques such as isotopic labeling, enrichment strategies, and noise-suppression algorithms help in distinguishing true signals from background interference.

Improving Throughput in Multi-Omics

Throughput in multi-omics refers to the number of samples or data points that can be analyzed simultaneously. High throughput is crucial for large-scale studies, clinical applications, and time-sensitive research projects.

Strategies to enhance throughput include:

Automation and Robotics: Automated systems streamline sample preparation, data acquisition, and analysis, drastically increasing the number of samples processed in parallel. Robotics also improve reproducibility and reduce human error.

Parallelization Techniques: Advances in multiplexing technologies allow multiple samples to be processed simultaneously.

For example, barcoding in sequencing enables the simultaneous analysis of hundreds of samples, while multiplexed tandem mass spectrometry enhances throughput in proteomics.

The Multi-Omics Revolution

High-Performance Computing (HPC): Multi-omics generates massive datasets, necessitating robust computational power. HPC systems and cloud-based platforms facilitate rapid data processing, enabling researchers to analyze large cohorts in less time.

Integration of Data Streams: Efficient data integration pipelines that combine omics data from multiple platforms streamline the analytical workflow. Tools like bioinformatics platforms and machine learning models automate the integration process, boosting throughput.

Overcoming Analytical Challenges

In addition to technical challenges, analytical hurdles must be addressed to improve sensitivity and throughput effectively.

These challenges include data complexity, variability, and integration across diverse omics layers.

Data Standardization: The variability in data formats across omics platforms is a significant challenge.

Standardized data formats and protocols enhance interoperability, facilitating seamless integration and analysis.

Quality Control and Normalization: Analytical sensitivity can be compromised by batch effects, technical variations, and experimental biases.

Rigorous quality control procedures and data normalization methods help ensure reliable and reproducible results.

Advanced Algorithms: Multi-omics data are inherently complex, requiring sophisticated algorithms for analysis.

Machine learning and artificial intelligence (AI) have emerged as powerful tools for identifying patterns, correlations, and causal relationships in high-dimensional data.

Scalability of Analytical Tools: To meet the demands of high-throughput studies, analytical tools must be scalable.

Cloud computing, distributed processing, and scalable software architectures enable efficient handling of large datasets without compromising performance.

Bridging Sensitivity and Throughput: The Path Forward

Achieving a balance between sensitivity and throughput is critical for the success of multi-omics studies. High sensitivity ensures the detection of biologically meaningful signals, while high throughput enables comprehensive and large-scale investigations.

Innovations in hardware, software, and methodologies are converging to address these dual needs.

Hybrid Approaches: Combining techniques such as single-cell omics with high-throughput methods provides the best of both worlds.

For instance, single-cell RNA sequencing (scRNA-seq) offers unparalleled sensitivity, while barcoding and parallel sequencing maintain throughput.

Collaborative Platforms: Open-source bioinformatics platforms and collaborative initiatives foster the development of tools that optimize both sensitivity and throughput. Collaborative frameworks also allow researchers to share data, reducing redundancy and accelerating innovation.

Future Prospects: Emerging technologies like quantum computing, nanotechnology-based sensors, and real-time sequencing hold immense potential for further improving sensitivity and throughput. As these technologies mature, they will revolutionize the multi-omics landscape.

The Multi-Omics Revolution

The multi-omics revolution is reshaping modern biology and medicine, but its success hinges on overcoming technical and analytical challenges. Improving sensitivity and throughput is central to this endeavor. By leveraging cutting-edge technologies, robust analytical methods, and collaborative efforts, researchers can unlock the full potential of multi-omics, paving the way for transformative discoveries and applications.

Handling Batch Effects and Noise

In the era of the multi-omics revolution, where data from genomics, transcriptomics, proteomics, metabolomics, and other omics fields are integrated to uncover deeper biological insights, technical challenges like batch effects and noise often stand as significant hurdles. Overcoming these challenges is critical for ensuring data reliability and drawing accurate biological conclusions.

Let's delve into these issues and explore strategies to address them in a clear, structured manner.

Understanding Batch Effects

Batch effects occur when technical variations, rather than biological differences, drive differences in datasets. These variations can arise from multiple sources, such as differences in reagent lots, sample preparation methods, laboratory instruments, or personnel performing the experiments. Batch effects can mask true biological signals or even generate false associations, leading to flawed interpretations.

For instance, in a proteomics study, variations in mass spectrometry calibration or reagent quality can create spurious differences between experimental groups. Similarly, in transcriptomics, RNA sequencing performed on different days or using different sequencing platforms can lead to variations that do not reflect actual gene expression changes.

The Role of Noise

Noise in multi-omics data refers to random variations or errors introduced during data collection, processing, and analysis.

Unlike batch effects, which are systematic, noise is unpredictable and can obscure subtle but important biological signals.

Noise can stem from instrument sensitivity, sample degradation, or stochastic biological variability.

This randomness makes it difficult to distinguish meaningful patterns from background fluctuations.

Strategies to Handle Batch Effects and Noise

1. Experimental Design
A robust experimental design is the first step in mitigating batch effects. Randomization of samples across batches, consistent use of reagents, and adherence to standardized protocols can help minimize systematic biases.

Including replicates for each condition and balancing sample groups across batches can further reduce the impact of batch-specific variations.

2. Normalization Techniques
Normalization adjusts data to reduce technical variability while preserving biological differences.

In transcriptomics, methods like transcripts per million (TPM) or reads per kilobase of transcript per million mapped reads (RPKM) are commonly used.

In proteomics, intensity-based absolute quantification (iBAQ) is a popular normalization method. Multi-omics integration platforms often include normalization steps to align data from different omics layers.

The Multi-Omics Revolution

3. Batch Correction Algorithms
Several statistical methods and algorithms can identify and correct batch effects. Principal component analysis (PCA) and hierarchical clustering help visualize batch effects. Tools like ComBat, part of the sva (surrogate variable analysis) package, use empirical Bayes frameworks to adjust for batch effects in high-dimensional datasets. For RNA sequencing, tools like limma and DESeq2 include batch correction options.

These methods systematically model batch-related variance and subtract it, leaving behind biologically meaningful variations.

4. Quality Control and Filtering
Quality control (QC) is essential for detecting and removing noisy or low-quality data. QC checks might include assessing sample integrity, ensuring proper alignment of sequencing reads, and evaluating missing values in proteomic or metabolomic data. Filtering out low-expression genes or low-abundance proteins reduces the noise level and focuses analysis on high-confidence data.

5. Use of Reference Controls
Including reference controls, such as spike-in standards or calibration samples, provides a baseline to distinguish technical variation from biological signals. These references allow researchers to monitor data consistency across batches and make necessary adjustments.

6. Machine Learning Approaches
Advanced machine learning methods can help manage batch effects and noise. Algorithms like batch effect removal with neural networks or random forests leverage complex patterns in the data to disentangle technical variability from biological information.

These approaches are especially powerful for multi-omics datasets where high dimensionality and interdependence between layers pose additional challenges.

7. Data Integration and Harmonization

Multi-omics studies often involve integrating data generated from various platforms and technologies.

Data harmonization approaches, such as canonical correlation analysis (CCA) and matrix factorization methods, align datasets while accounting for batch-specific differences.

These methods ensure that the combined data is coherent and interpretable.

Evaluating the Success of Correction Methods

Post-correction evaluation is crucial to assess the effectiveness of batch effect removal and noise reduction.

Techniques such as PCA, t-SNE (t-distributed stochastic neighbor embedding), and UMAP (uniform manifold approximation and projection) can visualize corrected datasets and ensure biological clusters are preserved while batch-driven separations are eliminated.

Challenges and Future Directions

Despite advances in batch effect correction and noise reduction, challenges remain. Correcting for batch effects without overfitting or introducing new biases is a delicate balance. Additionally, the lack of universal benchmarks for assessing correction methods complicates evaluation.

Future research is focused on developing more sophisticated algorithms that adapt to the unique complexities of multi-omics data.

The integration of standardized protocols, advanced statistical tools, and collaborative efforts to share best practices will be critical. As multi-omics technologies evolve, addressing batch effects and noise will remain central to maximizing the potential of this transformative scientific approach.

The Multi-Omics Revolution

Handling batch effects and noise in multi-omics data is essential for extracting meaningful biological insights.

By combining rigorous experimental design, robust statistical methods, and cutting-edge computational tools, researchers can overcome these challenges and unlock the full power of the multi-omics revolution.

Such efforts will pave the way for breakthroughs in understanding complex biological systems and advancing personalized medicine.

16. Ethical and Privacy Considerations

Handling Genetic Data from Single-Cell Studies

The rapid advancements in single-cell genomics have propelled our understanding of biology into a new era. By analyzing individual cells, scientists can unravel the complexity of tissues, trace the development of organisms, and identify subtle changes linked to diseases.

However, the collection, analysis, and storage of such detailed genetic data pose significant ethical and privacy challenges.

In the age of the multi-omics revolution, where various layers of biological data are integrated, addressing these issues becomes even more critical.

The Sensitivity of Single-Cell Data

Single-cell studies generate highly specific genetic data that can often be linked to an individual with extraordinary precision. Unlike bulk sequencing, which aggregates genetic information from multiple cells, single-cell techniques reveal the heterogeneity and uniqueness of each cell.

This granularity enhances the potential for biological discovery but simultaneously increases the risk of privacy breaches.

Genetic data inherently contains identifiable information, and the data from single-cell studies amplifies this risk due to the richness of detail. For example, single-cell sequencing may inadvertently reveal rare mutations that uniquely identify an individual or expose predispositions to diseases that the person may not wish to disclose.

Ethical Principles in Genetic Data Handling

Informed Consent
Before collecting genetic data, especially at the single-cell level, researchers must obtain informed consent from participants. Informed consent ensures individuals understand the scope of the study, the type of data being collected, and how it will be used. With single-cell studies, where findings may have unforeseen implications, it is crucial to clearly communicate potential risks, including privacy concerns and long-term implications.

Data Ownership and Control
Ethical handling of genetic data requires respecting participants' rights over their data. Participants should have the option to withdraw their data at any point, and researchers must establish protocols for securely removing the requested information from their databases.

Equity in Research
Single-cell studies often focus on populations with accessible genetic information, which could lead to biased outcomes that do not represent global diversity. Ethical frameworks must ensure inclusivity in research while protecting the privacy of marginalized groups who may face higher risks of misuse or discrimination.

Privacy Challenges and Strategies

Data De-identification
De-identification involves removing or masking personal identifiers from genetic data to prevent linking it back to the individual. However, with single-cell data, complete anonymization is challenging due to the high specificity of the information. Advanced statistical techniques, such as cryptographic hashing and differential privacy, can provide additional layers of protection by ensuring that individual data cannot be easily reconstructed.

Secure Data Storage and Access
Single-cell genetic data must be stored in secure databases with restricted access. Cloud-based platforms are often used for their scalability and efficiency, but they come with risks. Robust encryption and secure access protocols, such as multi-factor authentication, are essential to safeguard the data.

Researchers must also limit access to authorized personnel and monitor usage to prevent unauthorized sharing.

Data Sharing Frameworks
Collaborative research often requires data sharing, but sharing single-cell genetic data raises concerns about re-identification risks. To address this, researchers can employ controlled-access data repositories that enforce strict guidelines on who can access the data and for what purposes.

Additionally, data-sharing agreements should outline clear terms to prevent misuse.

Balancing Transparency and Privacy
While transparency in research is crucial for scientific progress, it should not compromise participant privacy. Publicly sharing aggregate results or summaries, rather than raw genetic data, is one way to strike this balance.

Researchers can also use synthetic datasets that mimic the original data's patterns without revealing actual information about individuals.

Legal and Social Implications
Governments and institutions must establish legal frameworks to regulate the collection, storage, and use of single-cell genetic data. Laws such as the General Data Protection Regulation (GDPR) in Europe and the Health Insurance Portability and Accountability Act (HIPAA) in the U.S. provide guidelines for protecting sensitive information. However, these laws need to evolve alongside technological advancements to address emerging challenges in single-cell genomics.

Moreover, societal perceptions play a significant role in shaping research practices. Public trust in science is critical, and researchers must actively engage communities to address concerns about genetic data misuse.

Transparent communication, community involvement, and stringent ethical oversight can help build confidence in single-cell studies and their potential benefits.

Looking Ahead: Ethical Innovation in the Multi-Omics Era

The integration of single-cell genomics with other omics data—such as transcriptomics, epigenomics, and proteomics—offers unparalleled insights into biological systems.

However, this also compounds ethical and privacy challenges, as combined datasets become even more revealing.

Researchers must adopt a proactive approach, embedding ethical considerations into every stage of study design and data analysis.

Emerging technologies, such as federated learning, may help by enabling collaborative analysis without centralizing sensitive data. Similarly, advances in artificial intelligence can aid in identifying privacy risks and optimizing data usage policies.

In conclusion, while single-cell genomics holds immense promise for understanding biology and improving human health, its ethical and privacy implications cannot be overlooked.

As we navigate the multi-omics revolution, a thoughtful and responsible approach to handling genetic data is essential to ensure that scientific progress benefits humanity without compromising individual rights.

17. Future Horizons in Single-Cell Multi-Omics

Potential Breakthroughs in Bioinformatics

Bioinformatics stands at the intersection of biology, computer science, and statistics, offering transformative tools to analyze and interpret the vast datasets generated by modern biological research.

The advent of multi-omics—a field that integrates diverse biological data types such as genomics, transcriptomics, proteomics, metabolomics, and epigenomics—has ushered in a new era of scientific discovery.

Here, we explore the potential breakthroughs in bioinformatics that are poised to revolutionize the way we understand biology and develop new medical and environmental solutions.

1. Integration of Multi-Omics Data

One of the most promising advancements in bioinformatics lies in the seamless integration of multi-omics data. Traditionally, researchers analyzed genomic or proteomic data in isolation, which provided a limited view of complex biological systems. With multi-omics approaches, bioinformatics now enables the synthesis of data from multiple layers of biology.

Advanced algorithms and machine learning models are being developed to unify these datasets, offering a comprehensive understanding of cellular processes, disease mechanisms, and environmental interactions.

This integration has immense potential for identifying novel biomarkers and therapeutic targets.

2. AI and Machine Learning in Data Analysis

Artificial intelligence (AI) and machine learning (ML) are revolutionizing bioinformatics by enabling the analysis of massive and complex biological datasets. These technologies can uncover hidden patterns, predict outcomes, and classify biological entities with unprecedented accuracy. For example, AI-driven models are being used to predict protein structures, simulate metabolic pathways, and identify drug candidates. In the multi-omics context, machine learning excels at deciphering relationships between various data types, such as linking genetic mutations with changes in protein function or metabolite levels.

3. Single-Cell Omics and Spatial Bioinformatics

Single-cell omics is a groundbreaking area that focuses on understanding cellular heterogeneity at an unprecedented resolution. By analyzing individual cells' genomics, transcriptomics, and proteomics, researchers can uncover unique cellular states and interactions within tissues. Spatial bioinformatics complements this by mapping these molecular profiles within their spatial context, revealing how cells interact in their native environments. These breakthroughs have vast implications for oncology, neuroscience, and developmental biology, offering insights into tumor microenvironments, brain connectivity, and organ formation.

4. Cloud Computing and Big Data Management

The sheer volume of data generated by multi-omics studies necessitates robust storage and processing solutions. Cloud computing has emerged as a game-changer, providing scalable and cost-effective platforms for bioinformatics analysis. These platforms enable real-time data sharing, collaboration, and high-throughput computations. Advanced data management strategies, such as FAIR (Findable, Accessible, Interoperable, and Reusable) principles, are ensuring that multi-omics data can be efficiently accessed and utilized across global research communities.

5. CRISPR and Bioinformatics Synergy

CRISPR-based gene editing has transformed genomics, and bioinformatics plays a pivotal role in guiding its application. Bioinformatics tools can predict off-target effects, design guide RNAs, and simulate the outcomes of genetic modifications. Coupling CRISPR technology with multi-omics data allows researchers to experimentally validate hypotheses derived from computational models.

This synergy is accelerating progress in gene therapy, functional genomics, and synthetic biology.

6. Predictive Medicine and Personalized Healthcare

Bioinformatics is enabling a shift from reactive to predictive medicine by integrating multi-omics data with patient health records. This approach allows for the identification of individuals at risk for specific diseases, early diagnosis, and tailored treatment plans. For example, multi-omics analyses can reveal how genetic variants influence drug metabolism, leading to personalized prescriptions that minimize side effects and maximize efficacy.

Such breakthroughs hold promise for combating complex diseases like cancer, diabetes, and neurodegenerative disorders.

7. Advances in Epigenomics

Epigenomics studies heritable changes in gene expression that do not involve alterations to the DNA sequence. Bioinformatics tools are essential for analyzing epigenomic data, such as DNA methylation patterns and histone modifications. Integrating epigenomic data with other omics layers provides insights into gene regulation, development, and disease progression.

This is particularly significant in understanding cancer epigenetics, where aberrant epigenetic marks drive tumor growth and resistance to therapy.

8. Synthetic Biology and Systems Bioinformatics

Synthetic biology involves designing and constructing biological systems with desired properties, often informed by bioinformatics insights. Systems bioinformatics models entire biological networks, predicting how genes, proteins, and metabolites interact within a system. These tools are vital for engineering microbes to produce biofuels, design novel biosensors, or develop new agricultural solutions. Combining synthetic biology with multi-omics data ensures precision and reliability in creating biologically engineered systems.

9. Microbiome Research and Metagenomics

The human microbiome and environmental microbiomes are vast reservoirs of genetic and metabolic information. Bioinformatics breakthroughs in metagenomics—analyzing genetic material recovered directly from environmental samples—are unlocking the potential of microbial communities. These insights are vital for understanding gut health, developing probiotics, and addressing environmental challenges such as bioremediation and carbon cycling.

10. Ethical and Computational Challenges

As bioinformatics drives forward the multi-omics revolution, ethical and computational challenges emerge. Managing sensitive patient data, ensuring equitable access to technologies, and addressing biases in algorithms are critical considerations. Furthermore, developing user-friendly tools that democratize bioinformatics for non-experts remains a priority.

In conclusion, bioinformatics is at the heart of the multi-omics revolution, bridging the gap between data and discovery. The potential breakthroughs in this field promise to reshape our understanding of biology, improve human health, and address global challenges with unparalleled precision and scope. The future is bright for bioinformatics as it continues to unravel the complexities of life, one dataset at a time.

Integrating Spatial Omics and Real-Time Analysis

The convergence of spatial omics and real-time analysis represents a groundbreaking shift in biological research, offering unprecedented insights into the complexity of living systems. Spatial omics refers to technologies that map the molecular profiles of cells in their native spatial context, while real-time analysis involves the immediate processing and interpretation of data as experiments unfold.

Together, these approaches are revolutionizing our ability to study biological systems with precision and speed.

Spatial Omics: A New Dimension of Understanding

Spatial omics technologies provide a detailed picture of how molecules, such as RNA, DNA, and proteins, are distributed within tissues and cells. Traditional omics approaches, like genomics and transcriptomics, offer a wealth of information about molecular content but lose spatial context by homogenizing samples. Spatial omics restores this dimension, allowing scientists to study the location-dependent behavior of molecules.

Technologies like spatial transcriptomics, imaging mass spectrometry, and spatial proteomics have enabled the visualization of molecular landscapes within tissues. For example, spatial transcriptomics combines high-resolution imaging with RNA sequencing to map gene expression across tissue sections. Similarly, imaging mass spectrometry captures the spatial distribution of metabolites and proteins.

These approaches help researchers unravel complex phenomena like tumor microenvironments, neural network activity, and developmental processes in exquisite detail.

Real-Time Analysis: Speed Meets Precision

Real-time analysis is transforming how we interpret biological data by offering immediate insights during experiments. This approach leverages powerful computational tools and machine learning algorithms to analyze data as it is collected. The ability to identify patterns, anomalies, and dynamic changes in real-time enhances experimental precision and adaptability.

In applications such as single-cell sequencing and live-cell imaging, real-time analysis allows scientists to track cellular behaviors, monitor physiological responses, and make adjustments on the fly. For instance, in precision medicine, real-time analysis can guide therapeutic interventions by rapidly analyzing a patient's molecular profile to identify optimal treatment strategies.

The Power of Integration

Integrating spatial omics with real-time analysis combines the strengths of both approaches, enabling dynamic, high-resolution exploration of molecular landscapes. This integration addresses key challenges in understanding cellular heterogeneity, temporal dynamics, and spatial organization.

For example, in cancer research, spatial omics can map the distribution of tumor cells, immune cells, and stromal components within a tumor. Real-time analysis can then interpret this data to identify cellular interactions, signaling pathways, and potential therapeutic targets. This integrated approach accelerates the discovery of biomarkers and facilitates the development of personalized treatment plans.

In neuroscience, the combination of spatial omics and real-time analysis provides insights into brain activity. Spatial transcriptomics can reveal gene expression patterns in specific brain regions, while real-time analysis of neural signals captures activity in response to stimuli. Together, these methods advance our understanding of brain function and disorders.

Enabling Technologies and Innovations

The integration of spatial omics and real-time analysis relies on advanced tools and methodologies. High-throughput sequencing technologies, multi-modal imaging systems, and machine learning algorithms are at the forefront of this revolution. Innovations in microfluidics and nanotechnology have further enhanced the sensitivity and scalability of these approaches.

One notable advancement is the development of computational pipelines capable of processing spatial omics data in real-time. These pipelines integrate imaging data with molecular sequencing outputs, enabling seamless interpretation.

Machine learning models trained on large datasets can predict molecular interactions, identify novel patterns, and generate hypotheses for further investigation.

Challenges and Future Directions

Despite its transformative potential, integrating spatial omics and real-time analysis presents several challenges. Data complexity is a significant hurdle, as spatial omics generates vast amounts of high-dimensional data. Developing efficient algorithms and scalable computational frameworks is essential to address this challenge.

Another obstacle is the need for standardized protocols and cross-platform compatibility. Harmonizing data from diverse spatial omics and real-time analysis platforms is critical for reproducibility and collaborative research.

Looking ahead, the integration of artificial intelligence (AI) with spatial omics and real-time analysis holds immense promise. AI-driven tools can enhance data interpretation, automate workflows, and uncover hidden insights.

The Multi-Omics Revolution

Additionally, advances in multiplexed imaging and single-cell technologies will further refine spatial resolution and analytical depth.

Transformative Applications

The integration of spatial omics and real-time analysis has far-reaching applications in medicine, biology, and beyond. In personalized medicine, these approaches enable precise diagnosis and treatment by mapping patient-specific molecular profiles.

In drug development, they accelerate target discovery and optimize therapeutic design.

Environmental science, agriculture, and synthetic biology also stand to benefit from these advancements.

As we harness the power of spatial omics and real-time analysis, the biological sciences are entering a new era of discovery.

By bridging spatial and temporal dimensions, this integrated approach provides a holistic view of life's complexity, paving the way for innovations that will reshape science and medicine in profound ways.

18. Revolutionizing Biology and Medicine

Summary of Transformative Impacts

The multi-omics revolution represents a groundbreaking leap in our ability to understand and manipulate biological systems. By integrating data from genomics, transcriptomics, proteomics, metabolomics, and other omics disciplines, multi-omics has unlocked a deeper, more interconnected view of life.

This transformative approach is reshaping fields as diverse as medicine, agriculture, environmental science, and biotechnology.

Here, we explore the profound impacts of the multi-omics revolution in ways that are accessible and relevant to everyday life.

1. Revolutionizing Healthcare: Precision Medicine

One of the most significant impacts of multi-omics is its contribution to precision medicine. By analyzing an individual's genetic code (genomics), RNA expression (transcriptomics), protein activity (proteomics), and metabolic profiles (metabolomics), researchers can create highly personalized treatment plans.

For instance, multi-omics analyses have revolutionized cancer treatment.

By identifying specific genetic mutations and metabolic signatures in tumors, oncologists can select therapies tailored to each patient, improving outcomes and reducing side effects.

The Multi-Omics Revolution

Multi-omics has also transformed the understanding and treatment of rare genetic disorders. Conditions once considered untreatable are now being managed or even cured through therapies developed using insights from integrated omics data. For example, gene-editing technologies like CRISPR were partly enabled by multi-omics studies, offering hope to patients with inherited diseases.

2. Accelerating Drug Development

The pharmaceutical industry has benefited immensely from the multi-omics revolution. Traditional drug development often relied on trial-and-error methods, which were time-consuming and expensive.

Multi-omics has changed this paradigm by providing detailed molecular insights into diseases. By identifying biomarkers — measurable indicators of a biological state or condition — researchers can streamline drug discovery and clinical trials.

For example, multi-omics has facilitated the identification of novel drug targets for diseases such as Alzheimer's, diabetes, and autoimmune disorders.

Combining data from various omics layers enables scientists to predict a drug's efficacy and potential side effects more accurately, thereby reducing the risk of late-stage failures.

3. Advancing Agricultural Science

In agriculture, multi-omics is driving innovations in crop and livestock improvement. Genomic sequencing of plants and animals, coupled with transcriptomics and metabolomics, allows researchers to identify traits linked to higher yields, disease resistance, or climate resilience.

This integrated approach is critical for addressing food security challenges in the face of a growing global population and climate change.

For instance, researchers are using multi-omics to develop crops that require less water or can thrive in saline soils. Similarly, multi-omics insights are improving animal breeding programs, leading to livestock with enhanced productivity and resistance to diseases.

4. Environmental Applications

The multi-omics revolution has also transformed our understanding of ecosystems and their intricate web of interactions. Environmental scientists use metagenomics — the study of genetic material recovered directly from environmental samples — to explore microbial communities in soil, water, and air.

When combined with proteomics and metabolomics, this approach reveals how microorganisms contribute to nutrient cycling, pollution breakdown, and ecosystem stability.

For example, multi-omics has been pivotal in identifying microbial species capable of breaking down plastics or cleaning up oil spills. Such insights are essential for developing sustainable solutions to environmental challenges.

5. Unraveling Complex Diseases

Complex diseases like diabetes, heart disease, and neurodegenerative disorders often arise from the interplay of multiple biological factors. Single-layer omics approaches, while valuable, often fall short in capturing this complexity. Multi-omics integration enables researchers to unravel the intricate networks of genes, proteins, and metabolites involved in these diseases.

For instance, in the study of neurodegenerative diseases like Parkinson's or Alzheimer's, multi-omics has provided insights into the underlying mechanisms, identifying potential therapeutic targets. This holistic understanding of disease pathways holds the promise of more effective interventions and preventative strategies.

6. Empowering Synthetic Biology

Synthetic biology — the design and engineering of biological systems — has gained momentum through multi-omics insights. By understanding how genes, proteins, and metabolites interact, scientists can design microbes to produce biofuels, biodegradable plastics, or pharmaceuticals.

For example, multi-omics approaches have been used to engineer yeast that produces artemisinin, a key antimalarial drug, in a cost-effective manner.

7. Improving Lifestyle and Wellness

Beyond its scientific applications, multi-omics is also influencing how individuals approach health and wellness. The burgeoning field of personalized nutrition, or "nutrigenomics," uses genomic and metabolomic data to tailor dietary recommendations. This approach helps individuals optimize their diets based on genetic predispositions and metabolic needs, promoting long-term health and wellness.

Additionally, wearable health technologies are increasingly integrating multi-omics data. These devices can provide users with real-time insights into their biological state, empowering them to make informed decisions about their health and lifestyle.

8. Transforming Research Practices

Multi-omics is not just a tool for specific applications; it is reshaping the very nature of scientific research. By promoting interdisciplinary collaboration among biologists, chemists, data scientists, and engineers, it fosters innovation and accelerates discovery. The integration of big data analytics and machine learning has been instrumental in handling the massive datasets generated by multi-omics studies, enabling researchers to draw meaningful conclusions with unprecedented speed and accuracy.

9. Future Horizons

The transformative impacts of the multi-omics revolution are only beginning to unfold. As technologies advance and data integration improves, the potential for new breakthroughs grows exponentially.

From combating pandemics to engineering sustainable bio-based industries, the applications of multi-omics are boundless.

The multi-omics revolution is more than a scientific advancement; it is a lens through which we are redefining our understanding of life. Its transformative impacts span healthcare, agriculture, environmental science, and beyond, offering solutions to some of humanity's most pressing challenges.

By embracing the power of multi-omics, we stand on the brink of a future where precision, sustainability, and innovation converge to improve lives worldwide.

Vision for the Next Decade in Single-Cell Multi-Omics

Single-cell multi-omics represents one of the most transformative scientific approaches in modern biology, allowing unprecedented insights into the complex interplay of molecular processes within individual cells. As we look to the next decade, the potential of this field is immense, promising breakthroughs in personalized medicine, systems biology, and beyond.

The vision for the future encompasses technological innovations, integration with artificial intelligence (AI), enhanced accessibility, and the unraveling of biological mysteries with precision and scale.

The Multi-Omics Revolution

Technological Advancements

The next decade will witness significant strides in the technologies underlying single-cell multi-omics. Current platforms, though revolutionary, face limitations in throughput, resolution, and cost. Advances in microfluidics, nanopore sequencing, and high-dimensional imaging are expected to overcome these barriers, enabling the analysis of millions of cells in parallel at a fraction of the current cost. Miniaturization and automation will also play pivotal roles, creating user-friendly platforms for widespread use in both research and clinical settings.

A crucial focus will be on improving the integration of different omics layers, such as genomics, transcriptomics, epigenomics, proteomics, and metabolomics. Current techniques often require separate workflows, leading to data fragmentation. In the coming years, the development of unified platforms capable of analyzing multiple layers simultaneously within the same cell will revolutionize our ability to construct comprehensive cellular profiles.

Integration with Artificial Intelligence

The sheer volume of data generated by single-cell multi-omics necessitates the use of advanced computational tools for meaningful interpretation. AI and machine learning (ML) are poised to become indispensable in this field. Over the next decade, algorithms will evolve to provide real-time insights, identifying patterns and predicting cellular behaviors with remarkable accuracy.

Furthermore, AI-driven tools will enable researchers to uncover hidden relationships between omics layers, revealing how genetic mutations influence protein networks or how epigenetic modifications affect metabolic pathways. This capability will be particularly transformative in understanding complex diseases such as cancer, where cellular heterogeneity often drives treatment resistance.

Applications in Precision Medicine

One of the most promising frontiers for single-cell multi-omics is its application in precision medicine. Over the next ten years, this approach will redefine how diseases are diagnosed, treated, and monitored.

By providing a detailed molecular blueprint of diseased and healthy cells, single-cell multi-omics will enable the development of highly personalized therapies tailored to an individual's unique cellular landscape.

In oncology, for instance, single-cell multi-omics could identify rare tumor cell populations responsible for metastasis or drug resistance, leading to more effective interventions.

Similarly, in autoimmune diseases, the technology could pinpoint the specific immune cell subtypes driving inflammation, enabling targeted treatments with fewer side effects.

Bridging Basic and Translational Research

The next decade will also see single-cell multi-omics bridging the gap between basic and translational research. By providing high-resolution insights into cellular processes, the technology will deepen our understanding of fundamental biology, such as cell differentiation, tissue development, and organogenesis.

These insights will directly inform regenerative medicine, where understanding the molecular cues that guide stem cell differentiation is critical for developing effective therapies.

In infectious diseases, single-cell multi-omics will shed light on host-pathogen interactions, identifying how specific pathogens hijack cellular machinery or evade immune responses.

These discoveries will be instrumental in developing novel vaccines and antimicrobial strategies.

The Multi-Omics Revolution

Accessibility and Democratization

To realize its full potential, single-cell multi-omics must become accessible to a broader range of researchers and clinicians. Currently, high costs and technical complexity restrict its use to specialized laboratories. Over the next decade, efforts to democratize this technology will be crucial.

Collaboration between academia, industry, and funding agencies will drive the development of cost-effective and user-friendly platforms. Educational initiatives will also play a vital role, equipping researchers and clinicians with the skills needed to harness the power of single-cell multi-omics.

Ethical and Regulatory Considerations

As the field progresses, ethical and regulatory frameworks will need to evolve to address the challenges associated with single-cell multi-omics. Issues such as data privacy, equitable access, and the responsible use of AI in data interpretation will require careful consideration. International collaboration will be essential to establish guidelines that ensure the ethical and equitable application of this transformative technology.

Tackling Grand Challenges

Looking ahead, single-cell multi-omics has the potential to address some of the grand challenges in biology and medicine. One such challenge is the creation of a comprehensive "cell atlas" that maps the molecular profiles of every cell type in the human body. This ambitious undertaking will provide an invaluable resource for understanding health and disease at an unprecedented level of detail.

Another grand challenge is the application of single-cell multi-omics to study aging. By revealing how molecular processes change within individual cells over time, the technology could uncover new strategies for promoting healthy aging and combating age-related diseases.

Collaboration and Interdisciplinary Efforts

The next decade will highlight the importance of interdisciplinary collaboration in advancing single-cell multi-omics. Biologists, bioinformaticians, engineers, and clinicians must work together to push the boundaries of what is possible.

International consortia and public-private partnerships will be instrumental in driving large-scale projects and ensuring that the benefits of single-cell multi-omics are shared globally.

The vision for the next decade in single-cell multi-omics is one of boundless potential. Through technological innovation, AI integration, and interdisciplinary collaboration, this field will continue to transform our understanding of biology and medicine.

By making single-cell multi-omics more accessible and applying it to tackle the most pressing challenges of our time, we stand on the brink of a revolution that will reshape science, healthcare, and society.

References

General Multi-Omics References

Hasin, Y., Seldin, M., & Lusis, A. (2017). Multi-omics approaches to disease. Genome Biology, 18(1), 83. https://doi.org/10.1186/s13059-017-1215-1

Li, X., & Lehner, B. (2013). Integrative multi-omics profiling: A holistic view of disease mechanisms. Nature Reviews Genetics, 14(7), 467-478. https://doi.org/10.1038/nrg3552

Wang, Z., Gerstein, M., & Snyder, M. (2009). RNA-Seq: A revolutionary tool for transcriptomics. Nature Reviews Genetics, 10(1), 57-63. https://doi.org/10.1038/nrg2484

Genomics References

Lander, E. S., & International Human Genome Sequencing Consortium. (2001). Initial sequencing and analysis of the human genome. Nature, 409(6822), 860-921. https://doi.org/10.1038/35057062

Venter, J. C., et al. (2001). The sequence of the human genome. Science, 291(5507), 1304-1351. https://doi.org/10.1126/science.1058040

Transcriptomics References

Mortazavi, A., Williams, B. A., McCue, K., Schaeffer, L., & Wold, B. (2008). Mapping and quantifying mammalian transcriptomes by RNA-Seq. Nature Methods, 5(7), 621-628. https://doi.org/10.1038/nmeth.1226

Stark, R., Grzelak, M., & Hadfield, J. (2019). RNA sequencing: The teenage years. Nature Reviews Genetics, 20(11), 631-656. https://doi.org/10.1038/s41576-019-0150-2

Proteomics References

Aebersold, R., & Mann, M. (2003). Mass spectrometry-based proteomics. Nature, 422(6928), 198-207. https://doi.org/10.1038/nature01511

Liu, Y., Buil, A., Collins, B. C., et al. (2017). Quantitative variation in proteome profiles reveals metabolic networks. Nature, 547(7661), 56-60. https://doi.org/10.1038/nature22358

Metabolomics References

Fiehn, O. (2002). Metabolomics: The link between genotypes and phenotypes. Plant Molecular Biology, 48(1-2), 155-171. https://doi.org/10.1023/A:1013713905833

Nicholson, J. K., Lindon, J. C., & Holmes, E. (1999). 'Metabonomics': Understanding the metabolic responses of living systems to pathophysiological stimuli via multivariate statistical analysis. Xenobiotica, 29(11), 1181-1189. https://doi.org/10.1080/004982599238047

Epigenomics References

Roadmap Epigenomics Consortium. (2015). Integrative analysis of 111 reference human epigenomes. Nature, 518(7539), 317-330. https://doi.org/10.1038/nature14248

Bird, A. (2007). Perceptions of epigenetics. Nature, 447(7143), 396-398. https://doi.org/10.1038/nature05913

Microbiomics References

Turnbaugh, P. J., et al. (2007). The human microbiome project. Nature, 449(7164), 804-810. https://doi.org/10.1038/nature06244

Gilbert, J. A., Blaser, M. J., Caporaso, J. G., et al. (2018). Current understanding of the human microbiome. Nature Medicine, 24(4), 392-400. https://doi.org/10.1038/nm.4517

Multi-Omics Integration References

Misra, B. B., & Langefeld, C. D. (2019). Integrative omics approaches for systems biology: Multi-omics and inter-omics networks. OMICS: A Journal of Integrative Biology, 23(11), 586-601. https://doi.org/10.1089/omi.2019.0134

Karczewski, K. J., & Snyder, M. P. (2018). Integrative omics for health and disease. Nature Reviews Genetics, 19(5), 299-310. https://doi.org/10.1038/nrg.2018.4

Systems Biology and Multi-Omics
Kitano, H. (2002). Computational systems biology. Nature, 420(6912), 206-210. https://doi.org/10.1038/nature01254

Auffray, C., Chen, Z., & Hood, L. (2009). Systems medicine: The future of medical genomics and healthcare. Genome Medicine, 1(1), 2. https://doi.org/10.1186/gm2

Technology and Computational Tools in Multi-Omics

Zhang, B., Wang, J., & Wang, X. (2019). Multi-omics data integration in cancer biology: Applications, challenges, and opportunities. Nature Reviews Cancer, 19(2), 91-107. https://doi.org/10.1038/s41568-018-0089-5

Libbrecht, M. W., & Noble, W. S. (2015). Machine learning applications in genetics and genomics. Nature Reviews Genetics, 16(6), 321-332. https://doi.org/10.1038/nrg3920

Genomics and Functional Genomics

Ramasamy, A., et al. (2014). A new approach to genotype imputation and association testing in low-coverage sequencing data sets. Nature Genetics, 46(4), 318-324. https://doi.org/10.1038/ng.2896

ENCODE Project Consortium. (2012). An integrated encyclopedia of DNA elements in the human genome. Nature, 489(7414), 57-74. https://doi.org/10.1038/nature11247

Transcriptomics

Wang, E. T., Sandberg, R., et al. (2008). Alternative isoform regulation in human tissue transcriptomes. Nature, 456(7221), 470-476. https://doi.org/10.1038/nature07509

Pertea, M., et al. (2016). Transcript-level expression analysis of RNA-seq experiments with HISAT, StringTie, and Ballgown. Nature Protocols, 11(9), 1650-1667. https://doi.org/10.1038/nprot.2016.095

Proteomics

Cox, J., & Mann, M. (2011). Quantitative, high-resolution proteomics for data-driven systems biology. Annual Review of Biochemistry, 80, 273-299. https://doi.org/10.1146/annurev-biochem-061308-093216

Nesvizhskii, A. I. (2014). Proteogenomics: Concepts, applications, and computational strategies. Nature Methods, 11(11), 1114-1125. https://doi.org/10.1038/nmeth.3144

Metabolomics

Kell, D. B., & Oliver, S. G. (2016). The metabolome 18 years on: A concept comes of age. Metabolomics, 12(9), 148. https://doi.org/10.1007/s11306-016-1108-4

Scalbert, A., et al. (2009). Metabolomics and genomics in personalized medicine: Towards a holistic understanding of the phenotype. Nature Reviews Genetics, 10(7), 491-503. https://doi.org/10.1038/nrg2623

Epigenomics

Jones, P. A., & Baylin, S. B. (2007). The epigenomics of cancer. Cell, 128(4), 683-692. https://doi.org/10.1016/j.cell.2007.01.029

Meissner, A., et al. (2008). Genome-scale DNA methylation maps of pluripotent and differentiated cells. Nature, 454(7205), 766-770. https://doi.org/10.1038/nature07107

Microbiomics

Qin, J., et al. (2010). A human gut microbial gene catalog established by metagenomic sequencing. Nature, 464(7285), 59-65. https://doi.org/10.1038/nature08821

Lozupone, C. A., Stombaugh, J., Gordon, J. I., Jansson, J. K., & Knight, R. (2012). Diversity, stability and resilience of the human gut microbiota. Nature, 489(7415), 220-230. https://doi.org/10.1038/nature11550

Multi-Omics and Systems Biology

Yugi, K., Kubota, H., Hatano, A., & Kuroda, S. (2016). Trans-omics: How to reconstruct biochemical networks across multiple omic layers. Nature Reviews Molecular Cell Biology, 17(12), 757-769. https://doi.org/10.1038/nrm.2016.137

Huang, S., Chaudhary, K., & Garmire, L. X. (2017). More is better: Recent progress in multi-omics data integration methods. Frontiers in Genetics, 8, 84. https://doi.org/10.3389/fgene.2017.00084

Case Studies and Practical Applications

Subramanian, I., Verma, S., Kumar, S., Jere, A., & Anamika, K. (2020). Multi-omics data integration, interpretation, and its application. Bioinformatics and Biology Insights, 14, 1-16. https://doi.org/10.1177/1177932219899051

Gross, S., & Agus, D. B. (2014). The emerging role of metabolic pathways in cancer therapy. Nature Reviews Cancer, 14(1), 11-22. https://doi.org/10.1038/nrc3867

Technologies and Computational Tools

Zhou, W., et al. (2019). Multi-omics profiling reveals widespread epigenomic and transcriptomic dysregulation in inflammatory bowel disease. Nature Communications, 10(1), 1-15. https://doi.org/10.1038/s41467-019-12326-1

Shamsaei, B., et al. (2020). A review of multi-omics data integration using deep learning. Frontiers in Genetics, 11, 570126. https://doi.org/10.3389/fgene.2020.570126

Future Directions in Multi-Omics

Torkamani, A., Andersen, K. G., Steinhubl, S. R., & Topol, E. J. (2017). High-definition medicine through omics. JAMA, 318(19), 1855-1856. https://doi.org/10.1001/jama.2017.15088

Yang, C., et al. (2020). Combining multi-omics data to investigate the complex human diseases. Briefings in Bioinformatics, 21(3), 649-663. https://doi.org/10.1093/bib/bbz111

General Multi-Omics and Integration

Zhou, X., et al. (2019). The next generation of multi-omics research: Applications and perspectives. Biological Reviews, 94(6), 1905-1923. https://doi.org/10.1111/brv.12534

Bersanelli, M., et al. (2016). Methods for the integration of multi-omics data: Mathematical aspects. BMC Bioinformatics, 17(2), 15-33. https://doi.org/10.1186/s12859-016-1161-9

Karczewski, K. J., & Franzosa, E. A. (2017). Multi-omics data integration in precision medicine. Current Opinion in Systems Biology, 2, 1-7. https://doi.org/10.1016/j.coisb.2017.01.004

Genomics and Population Studies

McCarroll, S. A., et al. (2008). Integrated detection and population-genetic analysis of SNPs and copy number variation. Nature Genetics, 40(10), 1166-1174. https://doi.org/10.1038/ng.238

Auton, A., & Abecasis, G. R. (2015). The 1000 Genomes Project Consortium: A global reference for human genetic variation. Nature, 526(7571), 68-74. https://doi.org/10.1038/nature15393

Transcriptomics: Novel Approaches

Trapnell, C., et al. (2012). Differential gene and transcript expression analysis of RNA-Seq experiments with TopHat and Cufflinks. Nature Protocols, 7(3), 562-578. https://doi.org/10.1038/nprot.2012.016

Stark, R., & Brown, G. (2020). RNA velocity: Predicting cell fate dynamics in single-cell RNA sequencing. Nature Methods, 17(9), 894-901. https://doi.org/10.1038/s41592-020-0865-y

Proteomics: Expanding Technologies

Wilhelm, M., et al. (2014). Mass-spectrometry-based draft of the human proteome. Nature, 509(7502), 582-587. https://doi.org/10.1038/nature13319

Huttlin, E. L., et al. (2015). The BioPlex Network: A systematic exploration of the human interactome. Cell, 162(2), 425-440. https://doi.org/10.1016/j.cell.2015.06.043

Metabolomics: Advanced Applications

Patti, G. J., Yanes, O., & Siuzdak, G. (2012). Innovation: Metabolomics: The apogee of the omics trilogy. Nature Reviews Molecular Cell Biology, 13(4), 263-269. https://doi.org/10.1038/nrm3314

Tsugawa, H., et al. (2019). A cheminformatics approach to characterize metabolomes in untargeted metabolomics. Nature Methods, 16(3), 295-298. https://doi.org/10.1038/s41592-019-0358-2

Epigenomics: Expanding Horizons

Smith, Z. D., & Meissner, A. (2013). DNA methylation: Roles in mammalian development. Nature Reviews Genetics, 14(3), 204-220. https://doi.org/10.1038/nrg3354

Reik, W., & Walter, J. (2001). Genomic imprinting: Parental influence on the genome. Nature Reviews Genetics, 2(1), 21-32. https://doi.org/10.1038/35047554

Microbiomics: New Frontiers

Faith, J. J., et al. (2013). Predicting a human gut microbiota's response to diet in gnotobiotic mice. Science, 341(6149), 1237439. https://doi.org/10.1126/science.1237439

Human Microbiome Project Consortium. (2019). A multi-omic perspective on host-microbiome interactions in IBD. Nature, 569(7758), 655-662. https://doi.org/10.1038/s41586-019-1237-9

Single-Cell Multi-Omics

Macaulay, I. C., & Voet, T. (2014). Single-cell genomics: Advances and future perspectives. PLoS Genetics, 10(1), e1004126. https://doi.org/10.1371/journal.pgen.1004126

Stuart, T., et al. (2019). Comprehensive integration of single-cell data. Cell, 177(7), 1888-1902.e21. https://doi.org/10.1016/j.cell.2019.05.031

Multi-Omics Integration Tools and Frameworks

Chen, S., & Zhang, L. (2021). Omics-evidence-based systems biology approach to precision medicine. Briefings in Bioinformatics, 22(3), 1-12. https://doi.org/10.1093/bib/bbz034

Argelaguet, R., et al. (2018). Multi-omics factor analysis: A framework for unsupervised integration of multi-omics data sets. Molecular Systems Biology, 14(6), e8124. https://doi.org/10.15252/msb.20178124

Applications in Precision Medicine

Kiyotani, K., et al. (2018). Multi-omics profiling for precision cancer medicine. Cancer Science, 109(3), 624-636. https://doi.org/10.1111/cas.13501

Hasnain, Z., et al. (2020). The multi-omics landscape of aggressive bladder cancer. Nature Reviews Urology, 17(8), 477-490. https://doi.org/10.1038/s41585-020-0320-5

Future Directions in Omics

Hood, L., & Friend, S. H. (2011). Predictive, personalized, preventive, and participatory (P4) cancer medicine. Nature Reviews Clinical Oncology, 8(3), 184-187. https://doi.org/10.1038/nrclinonc.2010.227

Wang, D., & Bodovitz, S. (2010). Single-cell analysis: The new frontier in 'omics.' Trends in Biotechnology, 28(6), 281-290. https://doi.org/10.1016/j.tibtech.2010.03.002

Multi-Omics and Big Data Integration

Hasin, Y., Seldin, M., & Lusis, A. (2017). Multi-omics approaches to disease. Genome Biology, 18(1), 83. https://doi.org/10.1186/s13059-017-1215-1

Wang, X., et al. (2014). Integration of multi-omics data for gene regulatory network inference and application to breast cancer. PLOS One, 9(2), e89398. https://doi.org/10.1371/journal.pone.0089398

Proteogenomics: Bridging Proteomics and Genomics

Aebersold, R., & Mann, M. (2016). Mass-spectrometry-based proteomics. Nature, 537(7620), 347-355. https://doi.org/10.1038/nature19949

Mertins, P., et al. (2016). Proteogenomics connects somatic mutations to signalling in breast cancer. Nature, 534(7605), 55-62. https://doi.org/10.1038/nature18003

Single-Cell Multi-Omics Advances

Clark, S. J., et al. (2018). Single-cell epigenomics: Powerful new methods for understanding gene regulation and cell identity. Genome Biology, 19(1), 72. https://doi.org/10.1186/s13059-018-1438-0

Argelaguet, R., et al. (2021). Deciphering cell fate decisions with single-cell multi-omics. Nature Reviews Genetics, 22(1), 67-88. https://doi.org/10.1038/s41576-020-00256-9

Metabolomics and Microbiomics

Tang, W. H., Wang, Z., & Levison, B. S. (2013). Intestinal microbiota metabolism of l-carnitine, a nutrient in red meat, promotes atherosclerosis. Nature Medicine, 19(5), 576-585. https://doi.org/10.1038/nm.3145

Mahieu, N. G., & Patti, G. J. (2017). Systems-level annotation of a metabolomics data set reduces 25,000 features to fewer than 1000 unique metabolites. Analytical Chemistry, 89(19), 10397-10406. https://doi.org/10.1021/acs.analchem.7b02323

Epigenomics and Environmental Influences

Rakyan, V. K., et al. (2011). Epigenome-wide association studies for common human diseases. Nature Reviews Genetics, 12(8), 529-541. https://doi.org/10.1038/nrg3000

Feil, R., & Fraga, M. F. (2012). Epigenetics and the environment: Emerging patterns and implications. Nature Reviews Genetics, 13(2), 97-109. https://doi.org/10.1038/nrg3142

Spatial Omics: A New Frontier

Liu, Y., et al. (2020). High-spatial-resolution multi-omics sequencing via deterministic barcoding in tissue. Cell, 183(6), 1665-1681. https://doi.org/10.1016/j.cell.2020.10.026

Stickels, R. R., et al. (2021). Highly sensitive spatial transcriptomics at near-cellular resolution with Slide-seqV2. Nature Biotechnology, 39(3), 313-319. https://doi.org/10.1038/s41587-020-0739-1

Integration of Omics in Agriculture

Luo, M. C., et al. (2009). A 4-gigabase physical map unlocks the structure and evolution of the complex genome of wheat. Nature, 457(7231), 431-436. https://doi.org/10.1038/nature07667

Bevan, M. W., et al. (2017). Genomic innovation for crop improvement. Nature, 543(7645), 346-354. https://doi.org/10.1038/nature22011

Neuro-Omics and Brain Research

Ecker, J. R., et al. (2017). The BRAIN Initiative: Mapping the dynamics of human brain cell types. Science, 358(6362), 690-691. https://doi.org/10.1126/science.aap8293

Khoury, N. M., et al. (2020). Epigenomic landscapes in Alzheimer's disease. Nature Neuroscience, 23(12), 1641-1652. https://doi.org/10.1038/s41593-020-00742-z

Paleogenomics and Evolutionary Studies

Prüfer, K., et al. (2014). The complete genome sequence of a Neanderthal from the Altai Mountains. Nature, 505(7481), 43-49. https://doi.org/10.1038/nature12886

Green, R. E., et al. (2010). A draft sequence of the Neandertal genome. Science, 328(5979), 710-722. https://doi.org/10.1126/science.1188021

Pharmaco-Omics: Personalized Medicine

Hood, L., & Flores, M. (2012). A personal view on systems medicine and the emergence of proactive P4 medicine: Predictive, preventive, personalized, and participatory. New Biotechnology, 29(6), 613-624. https://doi.org/10.1016/j.nbt.2012.03.004

Suhre, K., et al. (2011). Metabolic footprint of diabetes: A multiplatform metabolomics study in an epidemiological setting. PLOS One, 6(11), e23918.
https://doi.org/10.1371/journal.pone.0023918

Regulatory Frameworks for Omics Data

Mittelstadt, B. D., et al. (2016). Ethics of the health-related Internet of Things: A systematic review. Journal of Medical Internet Research, 18(2), e45.
https://doi.org/10.2196/jmir.5351

Fears, R., et al. (2014). Data access and sharing in omics research: Policy lessons from EU projects. Nature Reviews Genetics, 15(1), 7-15. https://doi.org/10.1038/nrg3624

Integration of Artificial Intelligence in Omics

Webb, S. (2018). Deep learning for biology. Nature, 554(7690), 555-557. https://doi.org/10.1038/d41586-018-02174-z

Angermueller, C., et al. (2016). Deep learning for computational biology. Molecular Systems Biology, 12(7), 878.
https://doi.org/10.15252/msb.20156651

Multi-Omics in Disease Modeling

Zhu, J., et al. (2012). Integrating large-scale functional genomic data to dissect the complexity of yeast regulatory networks. Nature Genetics, 44(8), 848-856.
https://doi.org/10.1038/ng.2311

Zolotareva, O., & Kleinewietfeld, M. (2019). Multi-omics approaches to study epigenetic modifications in autoimmune diseases. Clinical Epigenetics, 11(1), 81.
https://doi.org/10.1186/s13148-019-0670-6

Multi-Omics in Microbial Communities

HMP Consortium. (2012). Structure, function, and diversity of the healthy human microbiome. Nature, 486(7402), 207-214. https://doi.org/10.1038/nature11234

Anantharaman, K., et al. (2016). Thousands of microbial genomes shed light on interconnected biogeochemical processes in an aquifer system. Nature Communications, 7, 13219. https://doi.org/10.1038/ncomms13219

Epitranscriptomics and RNA Modifications

Dominissini, D., et al. (2012). Topology of the human and mouse m6A RNA methylomes revealed by m6A-seq. Nature, 485(7397), 201-206. https://doi.org/10.1038/nature11112

Meyer, K. D., & Jaffrey, S. R. (2017). Rethinking m6A readers, writers, and erasers. Annual Review of Cell and Developmental Biology, 33, 319-342. https://doi.org/10.1146/annurev-cellbio-100616-060758

Lipidomics and Its Integration in Multi-Omics

Quehenberger, O., & Dennis, E. A. (2011). The human plasma lipidome. New England Journal of Medicine, 365(19), 1812-1823. https://doi.org/10.1056/NEJMra1104901

Wenk, M. R. (2005). The emerging field of lipidomics. Nature Reviews Drug Discovery, 4(7), 594-610. https://doi.org/10.1038/nrd1776

Omics in Cancer Research
Weinstein, J. N., et al. (2013). The Cancer Genome Atlas Pan-Cancer analysis project. Nature Genetics, 45(10), 1113-1120. https://doi.org/10.1038/ng.2764

Zhang, B., et al. (2014). Proteogenomic characterization of human colon and rectal cancer. Nature, 513(7518), 382-387. https://doi.org/10.1038/nature13438

Multi-Omics in Plant Systems

Wu, A., et al. (2016). High-throughput sequencing reveals distinct small RNA landscapes in multiple ginseng tissues. Plant Journal, 85(3), 404-419. https://doi.org/10.1111/tpj.13099

Wang, W., et al. (2018). Multi-omics perspectives on wheat improvement under drought stress. Plant Biotechnology Journal, 16(4), 767-778. https://doi.org/10.1111/pbi.12884

Innovative Single-Cell Multi-Omics Techniques

Stuart, T., & Satija, R. (2019). Integrative single-cell analysis. Nature Reviews Genetics, 20(5), 257-272. https://doi.org/10.1038/s41576-019-0093-7

Zhu, C., et al. (2020). Joint profiling of histone modifications and transcriptome in single cells from mouse brain. Nature Methods, 17(8), 835-843. https://doi.org/10.1038/s41592-020-0881-7

Applications of Spatial Transcriptomics

Rodriques, S. G., et al. (2019). Slide-seq: A scalable technology for measuring genome-wide expression at high spatial resolution. Science, 363(6434), 1463-1467. https://doi.org/10.1126/science.aaw1219

Burgess, D. J. (2019). Spatial transcriptomics coming of age. Nature Reviews Genetics, 20(6), 317. https://doi.org/10.1038/s41576-019-0102-4

Bioinformatics and Computational Omics

Gentleman, R. C., et al. (2004). Bioconductor: Open software development for computational biology and bioinformatics. Genome Biology, 5(10), R80. https://doi.org/10.1186/gb-2004-5-10-r80

Bolger, A. M., Lohse, M., & Usadel, B. (2014). Trimmomatic: A flexible trimmer for Illumina sequence data. Bioinformatics, 30(15), 2114-2120. https://doi.org/10.1093/bioinformatics/btu170

Metagenomics and Functional Genomics

Qin, J., et al. (2010). A human gut microbial gene catalogue established by metagenomic sequencing. Nature, 464(7285), 59-65. https://doi.org/10.1038/nature08821

Sunagawa, S., et al. (2015). Structure and function of the global ocean microbiome. Science, 348(6237), 1261359. https://doi.org/10.1126/science.1261359

Regulatory and Ethical Considerations

Blasimme, A., & Vayena, E. (2020). The ethics of AI in biomedical research, patient care, and public health. Computational and Structural Biotechnology Journal, 18, 1287-1290. https://doi.org/10.1016/j.csbj.2020.06.013

Zwart, H., & Landeweerd, L. (2018). Multi-omics research, big data, and ethics. Science and Engineering Ethics, 24(3), 807-828. https://doi.org/10.1007/s11948-016-9782-1

Emerging Techniques in Multi-Omics Integration

Argelaguet, R., et al. (2018). Multi-Omics factor analysis—a framework for unsupervised integration of multi-omics data sets. Molecular Systems Biology, 14(6), e8124. https://doi.org/10.15252/msb.20178124

Meng, C., et al. (2016). Dimension reduction techniques for the integrative analysis of multi-omics data. Briefings in Bioinformatics, 17(4), 628-641. https://doi.org/10.1093/bib/bbv108

Multi-Omics in Precision Medicine

Hood, L., & Price, N. D. (2014). Demystifying disease, democratizing health care. Science Translational Medicine, 6(225), 225ed5. https://doi.org/10.1126/scitranslmed.3008604

Weston, A. D., & Hood, L. (2004). Systems biology, proteomics, and the future of health care: Toward predictive, preventive, and personalized medicine. Journal of Proteome Research, 3(2), 179-196. https://doi.org/10.1021/pr0499693

Proteomics and Phosphoproteomics

Sharma, K., et al. (2014). Ultradeep human phosphoproteome reveals a distinct regulatory nature of Tyr and Ser/Thr-based signaling. Cell Reports, 8(5), 1583-1594. https://doi.org/10.1016/j.celrep.2014.07.036

Mann, M., et al. (2013). Proteomic analysis of post-translational modifications. Nature Biotechnology, 31(11), 994-1005. https://doi.org/10.1038/nbt.2660

Metabolomics and Fluxomics

Patti, G. J., Yanes, O., & Siuzdak, G. (2012). Metabolomics: The apogee of the omics trilogy. Nature Reviews Molecular Cell Biology, 13(4), 263-269. https://doi.org/10.1038/nrm3314

Bordbar, A., et al. (2012). Personalized metabolic network modeling for assessing disease states and treatment outcomes. Nature Biotechnology, 30(9), 852-859. https://doi.org/10.1038/nbt.2344

Single-Cell Multi-Omics Advances

Darmanis, S., et al. (2015). A survey of human brain transcriptome diversity at the single-cell level. Proceedings of the National Academy of Sciences, 112(23), 7285-7290. https://doi.org/10.1073/pnas.1507125112

Macaulay, I. C., et al. (2015). G&T-seq: Parallel sequencing of single-cell genomes and transcriptomes. Nature Methods, 12(6), 519-522. https://doi.org/10.1038/nmeth.3370

Applications in Agricultural Genomics

Tardieu, F., et al. (2017). Plant phenomics, from sensors to knowledge. Current Biology, 27(15), R770-R783. https://doi.org/10.1016/j.cub.2017.05.055

Varshney, R. K., et al. (2019). Resequencing 429 chickpea accessions unravels genetic diversity and loci associated with agronomic traits. Nature Genetics, 51(5), 857-864. https://doi.org/10.1038/s41588-019-0401-3

Data Visualization and Analysis in Multi-Omics

Bostock, M., Ogievetsky, V., & Heer, J. (2011). D3: Data-driven documents. IEEE Transactions on Visualization and Computer Graphics, 17(12), 2301-2309. https://doi.org/10.1109/TVCG.2011.185

Gonzalez, A., et al. (2012). QIIME allows analysis of high-throughput community sequencing data. Nature Methods, 7(5), 335-336. https://doi.org/10.1038/nmeth.f.303

Multi-Omics in Epigenetics
Roadmap Epigenomics Consortium. (2015). Integrative analysis of 111 reference human epigenomes. Nature, 518(7539), 317-330. https://doi.org/10.1038/nature14248

Corces, M. R., et al. (2018). The chromatin accessibility landscape of primary human cancers. Science, 362(6413), eaav1898. https://doi.org/10.1126/science.aav1898

Microbiome Multi-Omics

Clemente, J. C., et al. (2012). The impact of the gut microbiota on human health: An integrative view. Cell, 148(6), 1258-1270. https://doi.org/10.1016/j.cell.2012.01.035

Lloyd-Price, J., et al. (2017). Multi-omics of the gut microbial ecosystem in inflammatory bowel diseases. Nature, 569(7758), 655-662. https://doi.org/10.1038/s41586-019-1237-9

Future of Multi-Omics in Healthcare

Mishra, S., et al. (2019). Multi-omics approaches to precision medicine in breast cancer. Nature Reviews Clinical Oncology, 16(7), 360-377.
https://doi.org/10.1038/s41571-019-0182-5

Yu, K. H., et al. (2016). Predicting non-small cell lung cancer prognosis by fully automated microscopic pathology image features. Nature Communications, 7, 12474.
https://doi.org/10.1038/ncomms12474

Innovations in Multi-Omics Platforms

Smolander, O. P., et al. (2019). Achievements of the Human Protein Atlas. Current Opinion in Structural Biology, 56, 129-134. https://doi.org/10.1016/j.sbi.2019.01.005

Ma, A., et al. (2020). A roadmap for translating multi-omics data into clinically useful information. Nature Biotechnology, 38(3), 293-295. https://doi.org/10.1038/s41587-020-0472-4

W J Francis

www.ingramcontent.com/pod-product-compliance
Lightning Source LLC
Chambersburg PA
CBHW071023240526
45469CB00006BD/2062